"Planning for your career can seem like a bad joke when you can't realistically plan for tomorrow...." The punch line is refreshingly hopeful, deeply realistic, and uniquely knowledgeable. I have read many chronic illness books. This one is very special. I was inspired to revisit fundamental issues related to my career plan, my outlook on life, and my responsibility to be my own ally and advocate.

> —Diana Murray, pancreatic and biliary disease,
> Associate Professor in Biological Sciences,
> Presbyterian Hospital, Columbia University.

Women, Work, and Autoimmune Disease tells stories that women (and men) can relate to and offers specific suggestions for how to live with chronic illness and not let it stop you. Too many people get stopped in their careers before they even have a chance to get going because of chronic illness. This book provides concrete examples and suggestions rather than the usual platitudes.

> —Art Mellor, multiple sclerosis,
> President, Accelerated Cure for MS

Rosalind Joffe and Joan Friedlander have created a much-needed field guide to navigating the workplace with a chronic illness. The book is clear, down-to-earth, and extraordinarily helpful.

> —Amy Tenderich, Journalist/Blogger,
> www. DiabetesMine.com. Author, *Know Your Numbers, Outlive Your Diabetes,*
> 2006 Winner, Lilly for Life Achievement Award for Diabetes Journalism

Rosalind and Joan are intimately aware of the extra complexity that having an autoimmune disease can introduce into one's life and work. Together they provide a roadmap for those facing such challenges, marked off with ample real-life stories, personal reflections, and sound professional advice. This book is a find for anyone looking for the motivational boost to keep working.

—Michelle Freshman MPH, MSN, APRN, BC, MSCN,
Newton-Wellesley Hospital Multiple Sclerosis
Clinic, Nurse Practitioner/Clinical Coordinator

Women, Work, and Autoimmune Disease is an invaluable support for workers with chronic diseases. Rosalind and Joan's insights and solutions based on experience are inspirational, easy to read and understand. The chapter on autoimmune diseases is the best explanation and categorization I have ever read. Rehab clinics would find this helpful to their own patients. It should be made available to employers, case managers, medical professionals and worker groups.

—Susan Iserhagen, PT, COO,
President DSI Work Solutions

Ladies, it's time to get out of bed and back to our lives. Rosalind and Joan have encouraged me to see the possibilities for reclaiming a dynamic career and helped me to believe these possibilities apply to me, despite my illness. My symptoms will be something I work around, not the only thing in my life.

—Sandy Lahmann, multiple sclerosis,
recipient of Adaptive Athlete of the Year award, 2007.

Any woman who struggles with chronic health problems needs to read this inspiring and empowering book. In a caring, straightforward style, Joan and Rosalind reveal how continuing to work can ultimately be the path to a healthier and happier life. *Women, Work, and Autoimmune Disease* will help you find the courage and strength to reclaim your career and your independence.

—C.J. Hayden, MCC
Author, *Get Clients Now!* and *Get Hired Now!*

Women, Work, and Autoimmune Disease

Keep Working, Girlfriend!

Rosalind Joffe, M.Ed.

and Joan Friedlander

EDITED BY L.G. MANSFIELD

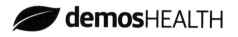 demosHEALTH

Visit our web site at www.demosmedpub.com

Medical information provided by Demos Health, in the absence of a visit with a health-care professional, must be considered as an educational service only. This book is not designed to replace a physician's independent judgment about the appropriateness or risks of a procedure or therapy for a given patient. Our purpose is to provide you with information that will help you make your own health-care decisions.

The information and opinions provided here are believed to be accurate and sound, based on the best judgment available to the authors, editors, and publisher, but readers who fail to consult appropriate health authorities assume the risk of any injuries. The publisher is not responsible for errors or omissions. The editors and publisher welcome any reader to report to the publisher any discrepancies or inaccuracies noticed.

SPECIAL DISCOUNTS ON BULK QUANTITIES of Demos Medical Publishing books are available to corporations, professional associations, pharmaceutical companies, healthcare organizations, and other qualifying groups. For details, please contact:

> Special Sales Department
> Demos Medical Publishing
> 386 Park Avenue South, Suite 301
> New York, NY 10016
> Phone: 800-532-8663 or 212-683-0072
> Fax: 212-683-0118
> E-mail: orderdept@demosmedpub.com

LIBRARY OF CONGRESS CATALOGING-IN-PUBLICATION DATA
Joffe, Rosalind.
  Women, Work, and Autoimmune Disease: Keep Working Girlfriend! / Rosalind Joffe, Joan Friedlander ; edited by L.G. Mansfield.
      p. cm.
  Includes index.
  ISBN-13: 978-1-932603-68-2 (pbk. : alk. paper)
  ISBN-10: 1-932603-68-9 (pbk. : alk. paper)
  1. Autoimmune diseases in women--Patients--Employment. I. Friedlander, Joan. II. Title.
  RC600.J64 2008
  362.196'978--dc22

                                                            2008001696

08 09 10   5 4 3 2

We dedicate this book
to the millions of women
who silently make their way
in the working world
while living with the effects of
a chronic and debilitating illness.

Contents

Acknowledgments

What would an acknowledgment be without first recognizing the people who live with us and love us? We thank our husbands, Jake Joffe and John Linzy, for their support through this painstaking, 2-year process—and for being thoughtful enough to leave us alone when we were struggling to meet deadlines. We are grateful to Rosalind's daughters, Lucy and EmmaRose, who offered useful comments that helped shape our ideas about what might appeal to "girlfriends," and always showed true grace in understanding when Mom was too busy to talk on the phone. And big hugs to Joan's son, Matt, for living his life on his own terms, and for being a part of a difficult journey.

This book would never have gotten past a rough draft if Elle Mansfield hadn't stepped in to allow our words to come alive and make sense out of the jumble. Elle's constant good humor and belief in this project helped us keep going when we weren't sure ourselves. And proofreader Cassandra Clark's knowledge of language and attention to detail assured us that we were true to the rules of grammar, syntax, and punctuation.

We also want to thank the people who have helped each of us make this happen: Jenni Prokopy of ChronicBabe.com, Michael Katz of Blue Penguin Development, C.J. Hayden of HowtoBecomeAHero.com, Janet Golden and the mentors who didn't know they were, and all of our clients who have taught us what it takes to keep working, girlfriend!

Authors' Note

If you've included this book in your reading list, you're most likely part of a sisterhood—an unconventional one, to be sure, but a sisterhood nevertheless. It's probably not a group you would ever choose to join, but that's one of the more generous components of autoimmune disease (AD): it's not exclusive.

You can be 10 or 50, Caucasian or Latina, a marathon runner or a couch potato. Although AD is wide ranging, it does have a preference for females between the ages of 25 and 40. What's more, it's partial to throwing the lives of those unsuspecting women into chaos, which is where the sisterhood comes into play.

We who have been blind-sided, tossed about, or even knocked down by AD have our stories to tell. These experiences are a rich mine of information that can serve as valuable tools for our sisters, helping to encourage and guide, to comfort and console. We have been placed on this circuitous path together, and together we can navigate its twists and turns, helping to ease the journey for each other.

In this book, you'll meet women who face challenges that are physical, emotional, intellectual, and spiritual. We have changed their names, but the heart of their stories remains unaltered. In each instance, these brave women have found ways to keep a strong sense of quality, satisfaction, and fulfillment in their lives. While the ways in which they have maintained their forward momentum differ, they share one fundamental decision: to stay in the workforce.

Their tales reflect their belief that continuing to be employed is a key element to health and well-being. In addition to boosting financial independence, employment stimulates the brain and fires the spirit. And let's not forget the sorry fact that once you're unemployed, it's harder to find a job.

Sure, working while living with AD can be difficult—trust us, we've both been through the "screw-work-I'm-gonna-stay-home" phase of our illnesses—once you move through the process a bit, you realize that you have a choice. You can remain stuck inside your head, preoccupied with your physical condition and your reliance on others for financial and emotional support. Or, you can reclaim your place in the bigger world, shifting your focus outside your body and participating in a community that is larger than One.

We believe it is far better to be part of the working world than to be a "sick person" at home. In our own experience, and from what other women have shared with us, work can play a positive and therapeutic role in the life of anyone who lives with chronic illness. All of the usual rewards that people derive from a job or career become even more important, because work can:

- Provide, or at least contribute to, financial self-support
- Connect you to other people around a common enterprise
- Focus your mind on external events, rather than solely on your health
- Offer challenges and rewards beyond your body's fluctuating health
- Allow you to be part of the "normal" world in the face of an abnormal situation

Whether you are coping with mildly debilitating symptoms or a disability that prevents you from doing what you once could, it is important to develop a long-term plan that affords you as much financial and emotional security as possible, while also allowing you to take care of your health. This is a very tall order, but one that is vital to your overall well-being.

Once you have identified the roadblocks to moving ahead, you can more easily break through them and determine those solutions that work best for you, your condition, and your situation. This takes strategic thinking: recognizing what you want, prioritizing your needs, and having the heart to go for it.

As we've said, it isn't easy. It requires adopting a "warrior spirit," which may be a new approach for you. The warrior rises above pain and fear, seeking solutions rather than falling victim. And there's another aspect to this battle: many of the women with whom we've spoken describe their awareness that illness can feel like both a curse and a blessing. Although they wouldn't have wished AD on themselves, they expressed gratitude for what they have learned and for the inner strength they have discovered as a result. It's the ultimate paradox.

We'd be willing to wager that your diagnosis of AD has meant that you may never view work the same way again and, at some point, you may need to make changes in how you go about doing your job. This book is intended to help you understand the decision points for designing a working life that supports your wellness—financially, mentally, and physically.

About the Authors

Rosalind Joffe, M.Ed., built on her own experience of working and living with chronic illnesses, including MS and ulcerative colitis, when she founded the career coaching firm, cicoach.com, dedicated to giving professionals with chronic illness the competencies they need 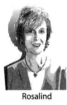 to succeed. She has held management positions in small businesses and a Fortune 500 company, and has taught in higher education. For more than thirty years, Rosalind has made decisions from a singular perspective: living with chronic illness does not preclude living a full life and workplace success.

Rosalind

Rosalind is a recognized national expert on chronic illness in the workplace. As a leading career coach, she has been quoted in *The Wall Street Journal, The Boston Globe, WebMD, ABC Radio, msnbc.com,* as well as a variety of regional and national media outlets. She writes her own eNewsletter/blog, WorkingWith ChronicIllness.com and together with Joan writes the blog, KeepWorkingGirlfriend.com. She has published in dozens of disease organization and health journals. She is a sought-after speaker and workshop leader for organizations that include the National Multiple Sclerosis Society, BiogenIdec, State Street Corporation, New Directions, Association of Career Professionals, HealthTalk.com, New England Arthritis Foundation, and the Scleroderma Association.

Rosalind holds a Masters in Education, is a certified Mediator, has completed training in Focusing Practice and the Corporate Coach University program, which is ICF accredited. She lives outside of Boston, MA with her husband. They have two grown daughters.

Joan Friedlander founded Lifework Business Partners, a national coaching and training company, in 2000. She has worked with hundreds of individuals in home-based service businesses, helping them to implement good business practices. Her focus is on guiding her clients to sustain themselves through the various stages of business growth, and to become more effective and comfortable with self-management, strategic planning, delegation and marketing.

Joan

Joan was diagnosed with Crohn's disease in 1992 and, with the exception of several short-term disability leaves, has successfully managed her career. In addition to coaching, she is a paid speaker, and has contributed to several published books, most recently the second edition of *Get Clients Now!* by C.J. Hayden, MCC.

Joan earned a B.A. degree in psychology from the University of California at Berkeley and is a graduate of Corporate Coach University. She is a recognized leader in her community, and has served on the board of the Orange County Chapter of the International Coach Federation for five years, including one as chapter president. She lives in Southern California with her husband; her son and step-sons live nearby.

Women,
Work, and
Autoimmune Disease

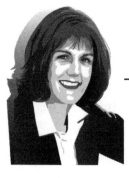

Joan

1

What Is an Autoimmune Disease, and Why Is It a Women's Issue?

The marketplace features a varied selection of books on the subject of women and autoimmune illness and, between us, Rosalind and I have probably read most of them. Abundant with information, they are a valuable resource, with a strong educational impact. We frequently cite them in this book—borrowing, extrapolating, and quoting from AD experts, because we are not trained in medicine and the corresponding disciplines. We are patients, like you, who are seeking to understand our illnesses.

Defining Autoimmune Illness

The medical community considers the majority of autoimmune illnesses to be chronic in nature. A *chronic illness* is one lasting 3 months or more, by the definition of the U.S. National Center for Health Statistics. Chronic illnesses, by nature, are longstanding problems with limited chance of recovery. A chronic illness may or may not cause visible impairment, limit activity, or require ongoing care; for most, no cure exists. Once autoimmunity is triggered, you are susceptible to recurrences for the rest of your life.

Autoimmune disease (AD) is further defined as an illness in which a person's immune system goes beyond its normal protective function, attacking the tissues or cells of a specific region of their own body. Something goes awry in the normal defense system, causing the body's immune system to turn on itself. Autoimmunity can affect almost any organ or body system—from skin cells to blood cells, from nerves to intestines, from joints to glands.

Because of AD's chronic nature, a correct diagnosis means that you should plan on dealing with the symptoms and necessary medication for the rest of your life. While it is possible to achieve remission—often for years at a time—the word "cure" is not yet part of the AD vocabulary.

Once an autoimmune disease is triggered, it seems to perpetuate a cycle. Unlike more common health challenges—such as colds and viral infections that can be treated and overcome—AD sticks around forever, even if it's not always active. This reality can be pretty horrifying, especially if you've been relatively healthy prior to the onset of symptoms.

A Sisterhood of Many

Experts have identified at least 63 distinct autoimmune illnesses. Yours is one of many that share similar characteristics (see the table for a list of all illnesses currently categorized as autoimmune). Some of the remaining 62 may be familiar to you, while others may seem completely alien and bizarre. There's certainly no need for you to have detailed information on those that do not affect you, but perhaps it will help you to know that, because of the broad scope of ADs, you really aren't alone...your co-worker in the cubicle down the hall or your boss's sister may have similar challenges.

Individually, each of the ADs are not very common—with the exception of lupus, rheumatoid arthritis, multiple sclerosis (MS), and scleroderma. However, viewed as a whole, ADs represent the fourth-largest cause of disability among women in the United States. According to the American Autoimmune Related

Autoimmune-Related Diseases

Alopecia areata	Ankylosing spondylitis	Antiphospholipid syndrome
Autoimmune Addison's disease	Autoimmune hemolytic anemia	Autoimmune-hepatitis
Autoimmune inner ear disease	Autoimmune lymphoproliferative syndrome (ALPS)	Autoimmune thrombocytopenic purpura (ATP)
Behçet's disease		Cardiomyopathy
Celiac sprue-dermatitis	Chronic fatigue syndrome immune deficiency syndrome (CFIDS)	Chronic inflammatory demyelinating polyneuropathy
Cicatricial pemphigoid	Cold agglutinin disease	CREST syndrome
Crohn's disease	Degos' disease	Dermatomyositis
Dermatomyositis—juvenile	Discoid lupus	Essential mixed cryoglobulinemia
Fibromyalgia—fibromyositis	Graves' disease	Guillain-Barré
Hashimoto's thyroiditis	Idiopathic pulmonary fibrosis	Idiopathic thrombocytopenia purpura (ITP)
IgA nephropathy	Insulin dependent diabetes (type I)	Juvenile arthritis
Lupus	Ménière's disease	Mixed connective tissue disease

Multiple sclerosis	Myasthenia gravis	Pemphigus vulgaris
Pernicious anemia	Polyarteritis nodosa	Polychondritis
Polyglandular syndromes	Polymyalgia rheumatica	Polymyositis and Dermatomyositis
Primary agamma-globulinemia	Primary biliary cirrhosis	Psoriasis
Raynaud's phenomenon	Reiter's syndrome	Rheumatic fever
Rheumatoid arthritis	Sarcoidosis	Scleroderma
Sjögren's syndrome	Stiff-man syn-drome	Takayasu arteritis
Temporal arteritis/ Giant cell arteritis	Ulcerative colitis	Uveitis

Diseases Association (AARDA), as many as 50 million Americans—20% of the population—are currently living with (although not necessarily disabled by) one of these chronic diseases.

Now, here's the kicker: the majority of autoimmune illnesses impact women more often than men. The ratios vary among the diseases from 2:1 to 50:1 (see table for statistics on specific AD illnesses). Some estimate that 75% of those affected—approximately 30 million people—are women. In light of these sta-

Female-to-Male Ratios in Autoimmune Diseases

Diseases	Female to Male Ratio
Hashimoto's disease/hypothyroiditis	50:1
Systemic lupus erythematosus	9:1
Sjögren's syndrome	9:1
Antiphospholipid syndrome	9:1
Primary biliary cirrhosis	9:1
Mixed connective tissue disease	8:1
Chronic active hepatitis	8:1
Graves' disease/hyperthyroiditis	7:1
Rheumatoid arthritis	4:1
Scleroderma	3:1
Myasthenia gravis	2:1
Multiple sclerosis	2:1
Chronic idiopathic thrombocytopenic purpura	2:1

Source: American Autoimmune Related Diseases Association.

tistics, it is surprising that autoimmunity is not widely regarded as a women's health issue.

Cause Unknown, Cure Undetermined

The initial concept of autoimmunity was discovered in the 1960s. Because this field of study is still so young, the causes of autoimmune illness are still unknown (and treatments are still in development stages), making diagnosis nearly as challenging as the illness itself. Clearly, much has been learned in 40 years. But because of AD's countless permutations, we are still a long way from easy diagnosis, full understanding, and comprehensive treatment. Furthermore, cures are almost never discussed.

When I was diagnosed with ulcerative colitis in 1992, it had not yet been definitively linked to the classifications of autoimmune illnesses. The first book I bought to further my understanding, *The Crohn's Disease and Ulcerative Colitis Fact Book*, was published in 1983 by the Crohn's and Colitis Foundation of America (1) and was touted as "the complete reference book for people with inflammatory bowel diseases (IBD)."

But as I read, I realized that a lot of guesswork was involved, and all possibilities were framed as questions. *Is it genetic? Could diet explain the differences?* At the time, experts were searching for a viral agent and a possible autoimmune response in those with IBD. Much has been clarified over the years, and the medicines I take today are different from those I took at first. What's more, after 5 years, a new symptom changed my initial diagnosis of ulcerative colitis to its sister inflammatory bowel affliction, Crohn's disease.

I imagine most physicians would agree on two primary observations: the medical profession has a lot to learn about autoimmune illnesses, and ADs are among the most difficult illnesses to diagnose and treat. Because research in this field is evolving and medicine is an imperfect science, it seems that autoimmunity is the most recent best guess for describing the causes of many conditions. In fact, it may be used as a catchall for those illnesses that are difficult to explain, and it may be diagnosed on assumptions and indirect evidence.

In time, scientists may find that this classification is quite different from our current understanding. For example, some researchers are raising questions about whether MS should be classified as an autoimmune illness. For our purposes, however, the discussion rests on how these illnesses affect a woman's life and how to best deal with them. Although each individual may experience a particular illness differently from another, many common concerns exist.

A Layperson's Explanation of Normal Immune Function

When your body is attacked—by a virus or a germ on a nail that you stepped on—your immune system goes into defense mode, identifying and killing anything that might cause you harm. If an infection persists or spreads, an *antibody* or cellular defense may be activated. These defenses, called *immune responses*, depend on the activation of white blood cells—the B and T lymphocytes—to provide protection against future infection.

The immune system is comprised of three layers, and each is engaged as the previous one fails to deal with the invasion:

Level 1: Skin and mucous membrane. Skin keeps foreign bodies out. Mucous membranes, including saliva and tears, contain enzymes that immediately go to work on invading foreign bodies.

Level 2: Innate immune system (neutrophils and macrophages). When we get a cut or a cold, the innate system launches a counterattack, generating inflammation. Macrophages, upon seeing an invader, attack to kill. They don't do a clean sweep, so other immune cells come in behind them. This can result in the pain associated with inflamed areas.

Level 3: Adaptive immune system. If a virus or bacteria penetrates the first two layers of the immune system and enters the bloodstream, macrophages sound the alarms to direct the activity of the adaptive immune system. As a result, white blood cells (lymphocytes) are sent out to search for the invader (*antigen*).

When the system does not work properly, this normal process can cause harm. Immune cells can mistake your body's own cells for invaders, attacking them in defense. This "friendly fire" can affect almost any part of the body, even many parts at once. Sometimes, an antigen—be it a virus, parasite, or bacteria—closely resembles healthy tissue, and the immune system unleashes antibodies against the foreign cells and mistakenly attacks and destroys healthy cells. Quite literally, the immune system turns on itself.

Why Things Go Awry

The latest research suggests that a combination of genetic markers and the right set of environmental factors will trigger the autoimmune response. If you have a certain gene or combination of genes, you are at risk for a particular AD, but you won't get the disease until something around you "turns on" your immune system. This could be a bacterial or viral infection, drugs, hormones, or something as seemingly benign as the sun or pregnancy. Amazingly, less than 10% of those who carry specific markers will actually get an autoimmune illness.

In many cases, once an autoimmune illness is activated, the body lacks the ability to return to homeostasis without medical interference, thereby generating the chronic diagnosis. However, it is important that we hold on to the hope that some combination of traditional medical treatments, allopathic remedies, and alternative therapies will result in a cure.

Present, Yet Undetected For Years

You may have signs of disease long before an acute flare-up of symptoms causes you to seek medical help. Many women, including Rosalind and me, can look back and recognize the signs years before the full onset of symptoms. The second time I was in the hospital, I spent a lot of time thinking about my body history. I realized that there may have been signs as early as my first months of life, and certainly by my teenage years, although I didn't have my first full-blown flare-up until I was 36.

Women—The Prime Autoimmune Disease Target

Current evidence suggests that women are exposed more often than men to possible AD triggers, primarily from the biological hormones and functions associated with the reproductive cycle. Think about it. We can carry babies in our wombs, even though half of that little being's DNA is foreign to our bodies. We must have some pretty interesting systems in place to prevent our bodies from engaging in full warfare on this partially "foreign object."

Another factor for women is estrogen, the hormone regulator. Estrogen can be a friendly hormone one day, then send things flying into imbalance on another. Researchers have discovered that symptoms of different illnesses—Crohn's, MS, and myasthenia gravis—may increase just before and during menstruation, when estrogen levels are higher. Interestingly enough, some diseases, such as Sjögren's syndrome, occur more often after menopause. And here you thought you had to worry only about the overt implications of the fluctuation of your periods!

It is vital, then, to engage in careful monitoring of the varying influences on your flare-ups and to learn to identify stressors.

As with everything else in life, nothing is universal and absolute. However, the trends and findings of recent years start to tell an interesting story. Autoimmune illnesses, chronic and unpredictable in nature, are a woman's issue and, as such, have serious ramifications for women in the workforce.

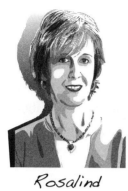

Rosalind

2

Why Should You Keep Working?

Sally lives with unremitting pain from chronic pancreatitis. Surgery hasn't solved the problem, and medication doesn't do a thorough job. Her position as a radiation therapist requires a high level of mental alertness and interaction with people, and Sally's medication leaves her feeling tired and mentally dull.

Her boss has supported her by allowing her to take time off when necessary. Although she feels better when she's not on her feet all day and can rest, it doesn't seem possible to take enough time off.

Sally finds that she resents the constant struggle to get through each day. She worries that if her boss leaves, a new supervisor might not be so supportive. She dreams of getting off the treadmill by quitting and taking disability. But the income wouldn't be enough for her and her two children to live on, and she fears that leaving her job would be a professional dead end. She is sadly resigned to the belief that continuing to work at her current job is the best option available, even if it isn't an easy one.

It doesn't take a lot of imagination to put yourself in Sally's shoes and see why she would fantasize about the day when she no longer has to work. In fact, it's been my experience that many women with chronic illness, particularly those with traditional jobs outside the home, seriously consider this option. Dreaming about the freedom to come and go on your own schedule and to not have to worry about disappointed co-workers or an angry boss when you can't meet a deadline seems enormously liberating.

And, of course, there are all those opportunities and luxuries you may never have had, such as exploring a new hobby, volunteering when you're well enough, napping when you want. Perhaps you could catch up on your reading, focus on your writing, take up painting. What a joy it would be to spend more time with your kids, go out to lunch with friends, or take a yoga class!

If quitting the workforce were to become a reality, the decision would most likely bring a strong sense of relief and even hopeful anticipation as you considered the possibilities. But as time marched on, these emotions might fade, replaced by an insidious fear that you would never be able to work again. This fear could expand into a feeling of being financially vulnerable, unable to support yourself without assistance ever again. Ultimately, it could lead to a sense of feeling trapped.

Wow! That's not a pretty picture. It's certainly not an inevitable outcome, but sadly, it's a common scenario. That's why we've written this book for those who are still employed but dream—innocently and perhaps inaccurately—about the alternative. We encourage you to keep working, girl friends.

Even Healthy Women Choose to Leave the Workforce

In her book *The Feminine Mistake: Are We Giving Up Too Much?*, author Leslie Bennetts (1) examines the habits of a "healthy" female population and discusses how motherhood can propel some women out of the workforce. From my reading of Bennetts, a woman makes this choice because:

- She believes that it's better for her family if she doesn't work.
- She believes that being a full-time mom and not working should be seen as a feminist option.
- She is unhappy in her career and sees quitting in the name of motherhood as a way out.

- The workplace is not amenable to part-time working mothers or high-powered-career working mothers.

These are just a few of the reasons that Bennetts cites to explain this phenomenon. And they are just as compelling for women with chronic illness, if not more so, because illness leaves less time and energy to divide between job and family.

For most women, child-rearing responsibilities demand a flexible work schedule, and the typical 40-hour work week is not necessarily the best fit. It can be difficult to find a well-paying, career-building position that offers the kind of schedule that many working mothers require.

Some women—particularly those with financial freedom or those who haven't invested heavily in career education—choose to stop working altogether for at least several years rather than face the juggling act of motherhood and working. Others might step off their career path and take a job with fewer responsibilities—and less pay.

Why Women should keep Working

Bennetts makes the case for women to keep working, regardless of their state of marital bliss or their sense of commitment to their children, because working is critical to their financial and mental well-being. Here, too, the rationale is equally sound for both "healthy" women and women with chronic illness:

- A salary puts food on the table, pays the rent, and hopefully provides decent health coverage.
- Work adds external structure to your day and gives you a place where you have to show up.
- It's not as easy as you might think to get back into the workforce once you climb out—certainly not at the same level as when you left.

The Addition of the Autoimmune Disease Component

Women who live with autoimmune disease (AD) must manage all these factors *and* their health challenges. Those who leave the workforce for several years, whether because of disability or child rearing, are in an even more precarious position because of AD issues. Disability might make it impossible to work full-time or to perform all the tasks of the jobs for which they are qualified. When competing for the few flexible jobs with applicants who don't have these limiting factors, women with AD often find that the scales do not tip in their favor.

Rosemary was diagnosed with Hashimoto's thyroiditis 1 year after giving birth to her third child. When she didn't feel well during her pregnancy, her doctor thought she was run down from having two children and a full-time job as a bank vice president. She didn't rally as quickly as she had after the other births, and when she returned to work, she was still very weak.

The diagnosis and the news that it was a treatable disease gave her hope that she'd get better quickly. But she hasn't responded well to the medication, and she continues to feel exhausted. Her husband wants her to resign from her job as vice president of client services for a regional bank—where she's worked since graduating from college—because he believes that quitting is the only way she's going to mend. When he asked Rosemary's doctor if working is hurting her health, the doctor replied that he honestly couldn't say for sure, but that the stress of working was probably not helping her.

What's more, Rosemary's mother has been sending her articles about how stress causes illness. Her best friend keeps asking her if she thinks she's being fair to her children. And Rosemary ignores them all.

She feels lucky to work for a company she likes, has

great benefits, and offers flexible scheduling. She finds that work is a respite from worrying about her health. And, most important, she believes that, in the long run, continuing to work will keep her healthier and happier.

Consider the perceived logic in the following statement: if work is stressful, and stress is harmful to those with AD, then work is harmful to mothers (and children). Even if you don't agree with this philosophy, your husband might. Your doctor might. And your mother most certainly does. The beliefs of those we respect can often lead us to do things we might not do on our accord—such as leaving the workplace against our better judgment. In my humble (but as you will learn in this book—emphatic) opinion, I believe this direction is the wrong one.

Looking at the Numbers

In 2005, nearly 60 million women were single or living without their husbands, compared to 57.5 million women living with a spouse. Comments William Frey, a demographer with the Brookings Institution, "For better or worse, women are less dependent on men or the institution of marriage (2)." Adds Sam

Roberts in an article entitled "51% of Women Are Now Living without a Spouse," "Younger women understand this better, and are preparing to live longer parts of their lives alone or with nonmarried partners. For many older boomer and senior women, the institution of marriage did not hold the promise they might have hoped for, growing up in an 'Ozzie and Harriet' era (3)."

The National Center for Health Statistics cites the divorce rate among the chronically ill as greater than 75%. Divorced women with children are already vulnerable to poverty, but divorced women with AD who do not have the means to support their families are even more susceptible. It's not a stretch to say that women can no longer rely on husbands to support them if they opt out of the workforce, for whatever reasons.

If that isn't enough to convince you that women with AD should keep working, read on.

The statistics regarding chronic illness and employment are striking. According to Partnership for Solutions, "An estimated 40% of the workforce has at least one chronic health condition, which they define as a medical problem that lasts a year or longer, limits what a person can do, and requires ongoing care. Twenty percent have two or more such conditions. And nearly 10 million American people work despite a disability (4)." The number of people with chronic illness in the workforce tells us that the issue is a clear and present factor.

The National Organization on Disability states, "Only 32% of Americans with disabilities [not just AD] aged 18 to 64 are working. But two-thirds of those unemployed would rather be working (5)."

Clearly, although many of us in the AD sisterhood struggle to stay employed, still others are unable to find a way to enter the workforce. Since 75% of those who live with an AD are women, and since AD comprises a large portion of chronic illness, AD undoubtedly plays a major role in the choices women make regarding their work life.

The Positive Aspects of Work

Statistics indicate that women should continue to work because they can no longer rely on men to provide financial support. But there are some other factors to take into consideration, as well.

Dina is a 52-year-old health writer who has lived with ulcerative colitis for almost 30 years. She has periodic flares and is increasingly debilitated by the disease, but she's thankful that it hasn't been a problem at work.

For most of her career, she worked for a newspaper. In addition, she rented a separate office with several friends so that she could spend time on her other writing projects. Last year, as the result of personnel reorganization and major cutbacks at the newspaper, Dina took an early retirement package.

Recently, two of the four people in her office decided they couldn't afford to continue to rent the space, so Dina opted to move her business into her home. Although her retirement benefits are sufficient, and she doesn't really have to work, she doesn't know what else to do with herself. Also, she's well aware that on days when she doesn't have meetings, she's likely to lie in bed and get depressed. She misses the camaraderie of working with others and the positive feedback of her peers, and she needs the social interaction more than she'd imagined. She's now thinking about finding office space to share with other freelancers.

Work is good for the spirit and your sense of self. It also gives structure to your day and occupies your mind so that you're not just thinking about your ailing body.

When I first started my business at home 10 years ago, I was still pretty sick from three surgeries (removal of my colon and an ileostomy) and the MS that was getting worse. Some days, I was so tired that I literally had to drag myself into the car to take my daughters to school. I'd often think that I should go back to bed rather than sit down to work in my home office. But I did work and, by lunchtime, I felt like a human being again.

Simply being productive always did the trick. I found that even on weekends, when I hadn't planned to work, I'd sit down at the computer when I was weary or out of sorts and quickly feel better. I noticed that while I didn't have a sense of physical improvement, I was pleasantly distracted and not so caught up in myself. And that was medicine that worked for me.

Now here's another statement to consider, and this one is supported by research: you will stay healthier if you continue to work.

Pamela, who has MS, always thought she would be a research scientist for the National Institute of Health. But she left research to teach at a university, because she loved working with students.

When her marriage dissolved, she was glad to have her work and her lab filled with graduate students to distract her. Her children were grown, and she was living on her own again for the first time in years. But when optic neu-

ritis recurred after 20 years, the other MS symptoms she'd been living with also became worse.

Within months, Pamela was bedridden and needed an aide in her home. She was only 45, but she felt as if she had transformed into an old woman overnight. Fearing that she would never be able to work again, she applied for disability—even though it meant selling her house and living on a much smaller income.

In time, her sister pointed out that Pamela was unusually depressed. Her daughter told her to go back to work.

Over the following months, Pamela's symptoms improved enough to enable her to get around on her own with a scooter, and she returned to work. Fortunately, her colleagues and students had kept things going in her absence, and she gradually got back into her work rhythm. She realized that she could use the scooter to move about the lab, and there were even days when her legs were strong enough for her to walk with a cane.

A recent United Kingdom study entitled "Is Work Good for Your Health and Well-Being?" showed that men and women who work have many health-related advantages over those who do not (6). This includes people with chronic illness, as long as the work they do is safe and accommodating. The findings state, "When their health conditions permit, sick and disabled people (particularly those with 'common health problems') could be encouraged and supported to remain in or to (re)-enter work as soon as possible because it:

- Is therapeutic
- Helps to promote recovery and rehabilitation
- Leads to better health outcomes
- Minimizes the harmful physical, mental, and social effects of long-term sickness absence
- Reduces poverty
- Improves quality of life and well-being"

"The Influence of Resources on Perceived Functional Limitations among Women with Multiple Sclerosis," a study by Evelyn Clingerman, Alexa Stuifbergen, and Heather Becker of the American Association of Neuroscience Nurses (7) suggests that women with MS have a better perception of themselves and their limitations when they continue to work.

The authors' research is based on the Conservation of Resources Theory (COR), originally presented in the article "Conservation of Resources: A New Attempt at Conceptualizing Stress" by S.E. Hobfoll (8). This theory proposes that various factors—including, but not limited to, money, knowledge, social support, and health—contribute to a person's well-being. The presence of one resource is linked to the existence of others; similarly, the lack of one resource is linked to the absence of others.

Given this concept, a woman with MS (or any AD) is more susceptible to a downward spiral because she lives with one less core resource: good health. Leaving the workforce because she thinks she can no longer do a job compounds her already lowered self-esteem. It's not hard to imagine that, if a person believes she is unable to do certain things, she is less likely to push herself to maintain social networks and physical health. Without the impetus to leave the house for work everyday, it's easy to become increasingly isolated and feel less than normal.

The study goes on to state, "Women with MS may be more affected by resource losses than other women, because of the challenges and stressors associated with their functional limitations. Hence, they may be more vulnerable to a loss spiral, in which their losses proliferate and escalate over time."

Another study entitled "The Quest for Ordinariness: Transition Experienced by Midlife Women Living with Chronic Illness" by D. Kralik found that with diagnosis and onset, there is an "extraordinary phase of turmoil and distress," followed by an "ordinary phase" that centers on developing the capacity to live with chronic illness (9). The researchers posed the question, "What is the meaning of living with chronic illness for midlife women?" They concluded, "Striving for ordinariness helped women to regain a sense of balance and control over their lives."

If we accept this information as valid, it is safe to conclude that many women with AD are in the extraordinary phase of their illness, while simultaneously developing careers and building families. As their relationship to illness moves into the ordinary phase, they seek ways to be just like everyone else, and a career can fill that need. If working is no longer a viable or satisfying option, it becomes much more difficult to regain that sense of ordinariness.

There's no doubt that exceptions exist to every rule. I know women with AD who have chosen not to work and do just fine. They don't regret their decision one iota. But such a scenario, although possible, is less probable in our current economic culture. I believe that women who live with AD are more likely to create the possibilities for long-term success and a satisfying and productive life when they continue to work. In my own experience and from the experiences of those with whom I've spoken, workplace success, in the face of illness, is transforming. It affords a sense

of personal power and confidence to face other challenges, large and small. And this is no mean feat.

Amen. Now, I'll get off the soapbox and give you
some concrete ideas about what I mean.

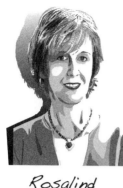

Rosalind

3

The Challenges of the Workplace

Chronic illness. Go ahead…it's okay if you shudder when you hear the words. Even though you've probably heard them a lot (and might think *What's wrong with me? I should be used to the sound and the meaning by now*), it's understandable that you still cringe. Let's face it—"chronic" means "ongoing," and the permanence (which doesn't mean that it's always present) of this condition can be very scary at first. But remember that the human spirit is amazingly resilient. You really can learn to cope.

Judy is 34, with a husband, two children, and a demanding job as a supervisor in the finance division of a large insurance company. When she was diagnosed with multiple sclerosis (MS) 6 years ago, her greatest struggle was with the unpredictability of her disease. Always a highly orga-

nized person, she would take to her bed each time a new or recurrent symptom flared—not because she couldn't keep going physically, but because she lost her will to move. Her life felt out of control, and she hated it.

After a day of lying in bed and crying (her husband would simply close the door and take over), Judy could pull herself together enough to manage the minimum. Her symptoms would eventually recede—sometimes after a few weeks and sometimes after several months—leaving her feeling like herself again.

When her boss told her that her performance was slipping, Judy realized that she had to do a better job of managing the unpredictability of her illness. With professional help, she came to a more accepting place about the changes in her body and her life. She worked with a coach, who helped her develop new skills that allowed her to fulfill her responsibilities, even when her body wasn't functioning at top performance. She wasn't happy about living with MS, but at least she could keep her job.

Take a moment to think about other, more benign changes that have taken place in your life over the years. Maybe you have stretch marks. Gray hairs or adult acne. An extra 20 pounds that resist every known diet and exercise plan. Perhaps each event upset you at first. But odds are you eventually said "Oh, big deal," and didn't allow these relatively minor maladies to take on exaggerated significance.

Now consider the more serious difficulties that you've faced. Separation or divorce. A child with emotional problems. The death of a parent. Just as the pain in your heart has eased and you have adapted, so, too, can you reach your peace with autoimmune disease (AD).

You might want to look upon this as one of the many unforeseen events that enter a person's world. Acceptance—regarding your illness, the unexpected, and your life—is often the first step toward gaining (or regaining) your sense of balance in the world. You can't control whether or not you develop a chronic illness. But you do have the power to confront and manage the challenges you face with AD. And, believe it or not, one place where you can do this is in the workplace. Although physical symptoms may wax and wane, you can develop greater control over your life. In fact, you can achieve mastery in the face of uncertainty.

Finding Your Internal Balance

We've all experienced the disappointment of not being able to do something that really matters to us because we are too sick. My first recollection of this was when I was

8 years old and contracted a virus that left me too sick to join my family and relatives for our Thanksgiving Day dinner. I vividly recall the keen sense of disappointment and, to my young mind, it seemed as if my world had collapsed. Fortunately, that illness didn't last, and bad health didn't cause me to miss anything again for a long time.

But in my late twenties, I developed MS. I learned the hard way that missing events and not being able to meet commitments can become an unpleasant fact of life. There's no getting around that when you live with a chronic illness. Either you accept it, or it wears you out.

Because AD symptoms can get worse and better—appearing out of the blue and disappearing just as quickly—it's impossible to predict what next week will be like, never mind tomorrow. Symptoms can prevent you from taking part in activities that are critical to your livelihood or that fire your passion. In my case, my love for skiing wasn't a problem with MS, but ulcerative colitis made it tough when I couldn't find a bathroom on the mountain.

Depending on your particular disease, you might always have the same symptoms, with variations in intensity and duration. For instance, your hands might be chronically stiff from scleroderma, but there can be moments, days, and even months when you barely notice it—and conversely, you may have periods when you are unable to use your hands at all.

Autoimmune diseases can randomly affect different parts of the body, in no particular order, with no rhyme or reason, and with no clear trigger, making it difficult to get a good handle on your life. Lupus might make it difficult to walk the stairs of your office building for several months. Then, a year later, you can walk just fine, but your painful hands make it difficult to carry a briefcase. And then you start having trouble finding words. Some people experience varying symptoms that come and go within a 12-hour period!

When you're confronted with your body's rollercoaster ride through your illness, you face not only your own reactions, but also those of people around you. For some, the responses of others are even more difficult to manage than their own. Let's face it: by nature, women are nurturing and helping beings, and it's troubling to disappoint others or fail to meet their expectations.

Saying "I can't" will probably never be easy, but it can become part of your repertoire and help to develop your sense of balance.

While we're on the subject, you've probably heard a lot of talk about "leading a balanced life." Typically, that refers to your external life—such as making time for family, exercising, and eating right. But "being in balance" refers to your internal metrics, enabling you to be resilient in the face of change and unpredictability.

Grace, a paralegal, loves to go to the park on weekends with her husband and their two small children. She dreads the days when she has to tell her family that she can't go with them because her headaches—a symptom of lupus— are so bad. She knows they'll feel let down, but she fears that if she pushes herself, she'll be unable to do anything else the rest of the weekend.

Begging off from a promise or responsibility is not an easy decision to make. My strategy has been to think about the pros and cons of each opportunity— and yes, these challenges are also opportunities—with the intention of saying yes whenever possible.

Meri, a human resources trainer, is supposed to lead a week-long off-site retreat for a client's senior team, but she very reluctantly turns over the bulk of the work to subordinates. The client specifically requested her, and she knows he'll be upset. But the Crohn's disease is making her too ill to stand in front of the group for extended periods of time.

Many times over the years, I couldn't attend a function or perform an activity that I had planned, and it's always difficult to experience the letdown yet again. And it never gets any easier to hear that I've disappointed others. But I've learned that I get more emotional—and even physical—strength from believing in the possibility than from limiting myself.

When Janet, who works in instructional technology support, was diagnosed with Crohn's disease at age 32, she cut out all nonessential activities from her work and home life. She never liked taking risks, and figured it was better to be safe than sorry. She stopped going to professional activities, no longer took on additional assignments, and chose not to participate in career-advancement training.

On the personal front, she and her husband made the difficult decision to postpone having children. But when her mother died suddenly and unexpectedly, Janet had a change of heart—and vision—about her life. She told her husband that they shouldn't wait to have children, and she signed up for a program at work that would increase her options.

Now, 15 years later, Janet has two children, works a reduced schedule, and feels good about the balance she's achieved. She purposefully explores new opportunities with optimism and with care. She has discovered that she is much happier taking the approach that she'll do it if she can and

live with the possibility of disappointment, rather than taking no risk at all. This is her sense of balance.

Remaining Stronger Than the Fear

*Amy was 26 when she collapsed after taking a hot shower
and was found unconscious several hours later. An MRI
showed that she had MS. When she read online about the
disease and its symptoms, she was shocked to discover that
she had probably been living with the disease for several
years without knowing it. She also read that people with
MS have to be careful not to get too tired or too stressed.
Her job as a stock analyst was both.*

*Terrified about losing consciousness again, she quit her
job and lived on her savings, doing very little other than
taking yoga classes and seeing friends. When she ran out
of money, she moved back in with her parents. After a few
months, her father told her that she looked fine and should get
a job. Amy knew that she wasn't fine, even if she appeared so
to her dad. Didn't he realize she had MS?*

*But Amy acknowledged that she was miserable.
Although she'd been healthy while not working and was
afraid to rock the boat, she missed her life, her job, and her
independence—a lot. Fortunately, her former boss called to
say that her old job was available, and it was hers if she
wanted it. She decided that working was her best bet for*

now. She had to stop being scared of what might happen and start living her life again.

Each of us is programmed with a level of denial that allows us to ignore the bad things that could happen in a lifetime. Without this defense mechanism, we probably wouldn't ever get out of bed in the morning:

> *I might be in a car accident.*
> *Today could be the day of the big earthquake.*
> *My house could get burglarized while I'm gone.*
> *I might be abducted by aliens.*

But thanks to these "denial microchips," we keep the fear of danger at bay, tucked away in our subconscious and unable to immobilize us. The relationship between children and parents provides a good example of how modest levels of denial work to our advantage. Most parents have no fear for themselves regarding illness and death, yet they are vigilant about protecting their offspring. Children, especially as they grow up, are equally determined to ignore or override that protection. Like their parents, their denial microchips are in full force regarding their own safety, and they can't believe that anything bad could happen to them. Somehow, we learn to live with these opposing forces.

However, when you experience disabling symptoms that leave you feeling like you're 70 when you're 25, you know that the unexpected and the ugly *do* happen. And suddenly, the strength of those denial chips gets weaker. Although everyone faces the reality that bad things happen to good people, you know that the likelihood is greater for you.

And that, girlfriend, leaves you with three choices: you can become paralyzed by fear, you can try to insulate yourself behind a protective barrier, or you can be catalyzed into thoughtful and productive action. Obviously, the first two responses are not going to help you live well with your disease. That leaves the third as the only option that allows you to continue to grow.

Identity, Productivity, and Delivery

Linda was 24 and considering law school when she was diagnosed with rheumatoid arthritis (RA). Always a high achiever, she decided that a law degree would guarantee a job, regardless of her health. When she graduated and was hired by a large firm, she disclosed her RA. It wasn't a factor in what she could do, and no one paid any attention to it—including Linda.

From the start, she sought the tough cases and extra assignments, because that's what she thrived on. She didn't want to refuse anything—nor did she think she should.

Shortly after giving birth to her second child, Linda experienced a dramatic increase in symptoms—not an uncommon occurrence among AD diseases. Five years later, her hands were less usable, making writing and word processing extremely difficult, and her joint problems required a hip operation. When she returned to work after the surgery, she was more driven than ever not to let her health get in her way.

After 15 years at the firm, Linda needed a second hip operation. Over the previous 2 years, she'd missed several important client meetings due to doctors' appointments and tests, and she required additional administrative help to compensate for her poorly functioning legs and hands. Her billable hours had dropped, threatening both her income and her position with the firm. No longer given coveted tasks, Linda believed that she was perceived as a less significant player. When she returned from surgery leave, the managing partner suggested that she cut back on her hours and take fewer cases and more administrative work. Linda was appalled and depressed.

In the twenty-first-century workplace, you are what you produce and what you deliver. For this reason alone, you have to be able to honestly assess your capabilities so that you can meet expectations—both yours and those of others. If you have a good work history, people will cut you slack if you falter now and then—but only for so long. It's up to you to figure out what you have to do to ensure that you continue to produce what people expect, and deliver it in the way they want it.

Fortunately, Linda's second hip-replacement surgery was successful, and she was able to walk normally again. New drugs succeeded in quieting her symptoms. More important, she gave herself time to readjust how she thinks about her health and her work.

She recognized that she had to make changes in her activities and schedule to fit her disabilities, so she decided to plan her future based on the current condition of her illness and its requirements. She realized that she might get better or worse, with no guarantees, but at least she could behave based on the reality of the situation, rather than on wishful thinking. She has cut her litigation practice by 50%, and has taken on more management responsibilities. She has told her partners that she will evaluate her position in 5 years to determine if she is still happy in her new role.

Linda has learned to respect her comfort level and create her own road map. She is a woman mastering both her sense of balance and the art of being responsible for what she can control.

Managing Your Work and Your Physical Health

To be sure, even healthy people struggle with the negative stress that comes from putting in too many hours at work, racing to meet tight deadlines, and not having the time to take breaks in the day to relax and regroup. When you live with AD, your body is already stressed, requiring even more tender loving care.

For Susan, a supervisor in a large school-system payroll office, numbers and deadlines are part of the job. On most days, her symptoms of fibromyalgia are relatively mild—periodic pain in her legs and fingers—but recently she's had several bad flares that have resulted in her need to take a leave from work. Her husband tells her angrily that if she took better care of herself, she wouldn't get sick.

But Susan isn't sure what makes her sick, so she ends up worrying about everything she does. She's discovering that she feels particularly bad when she's up against deadlines, but she doesn't see any way to avoid the tension.

Unassertive by nature, Susan carries the load when time crunches come up, because it's difficult for her to ask for help. This means that she works late and doesn't get enough sleep, leaving her feeling wiped out. When she recently took a time-management course, it helped her see that a bit of job-function tweaking and staff cross-training could help ease the pressure.

Although tight deadlines will probably always be a source of tension for her, they're part of her job. But Susan is mastering her ability to manage the things she can control.

Autoimmune diseases are fickle, and what might adversely impact your symptoms one day might not affect you the next. Some ADs are aggravated by tension and lack of sleep, while others are triggered by what you eat or the temperature of the room.

In general, people with ADs are advised to take better care of themselves. But how do you know what that means for you? Unfortunately, you won't find a roadmap or a GPS system to help you navigate this terrain. It's trial and error until you learn how your body responds to certain stimuli. And, as we well know, even that can shift, seemingly with the wind.

It is especially difficult to take thoughtful care of your health when your presence is required at a certain time on a certain day—and the new medication is creating intestinal problems. Or if you have to get the report done when you really need to sleep. Or when you have to walk long distances and your legs feel like logs. This becomes even more confusing when you felt fine working on a project 15 hours a day for 3 weeks running, but a few months later, you get a migraine after just two late-night meetings.

It's easy to fall into the habit of blaming yourself when you feel worse after pushing yourself. Playing Monday-morning quarterback, you assume that if you hadn't done that activity or worked so hard, you'd be fine now. Although you might think that you're teaching yourself a lesson by doing this, it's actually a waste of your time and precious resources. Instead, use these situations as an opportunity to learn about yourself and your health. Notice the questions in the sidebar. While they don't solve the situation, they'll help you create the mental model you need to develop mastery in living with the unpredictable.

When we're young, we dream about what we will be when we grow up. Sometimes, those dreams become reality. Other times, we make new plans based on who we've actually become. We can do that because we have confidence, based on experience, in our future. And it's still possible to do that again, even when you're facing AD's uncertain path.

◇◇◇◇◇◇◇◇◇◇◇◇◇◇◇◇◇◇◇◇◇◇◇◇◇◇◇◇◇◇◇◇◇◇◇◇

When You Want to Develop Mastery in Living with the Unpredictable

Ask Yourself:

- What is best for my mental and physical health when a problem situation comes up, given that I can't be sure how anything affects me?
- What can I do to change the workflow so it can be more balanced and I don't face these issues as frequently?
- How can I create more flexibility in my schedule?

Maureen has lived with chronic fatigue syndrome for 4 years. A researcher in a large bank, she's taken one short-term disability leave. But, for the most part, she manages her workload, even when she's not feeling up to snuff.

During her annual review, her boss told her that she's overqualified for the work, and asked if she's getting bored after 8 years. He suggested that she apply for the supervisor's job opening in the department. Alternatively, she might consider getting additional training and applying for a job in another department, where she would have more opportunities for career advancement. Maureen was stunned. Unable to imagine leaving what felt comfortable given her bad health, she also knew that she was bored and could use more money.

Planning for your career can seem like a bad joke when you can't realistically plan for tomorrow, but unpredictability makes it even more important for you to take charge. You, more than most people, know that plans must survive the test of flexibility. If you don't plan for what's possible, you're leaving it up to chance—and that creates a victim mentality.

After several months, Maureen sought help from a career counselor who understood her health issues. This allowed her to realistically explore both the pros and cons of taking a more proactive approach to her career. She decided not to take a supervisor's job, because she didn't want to be responsible for others with her fluctuating health. Instead, she opted to get additional training and apply for a different job that offered more variation and advancement potential.

Many organizations and even higher-education institutions offer career-development programs that help you determine what it takes to move forward in your chosen field. That's a good start. But you'll need to tweak the model to fit your health limitations and capitalize on your strengths. It takes clear-sighted focus and determination to make this work for you.

Trying Something New

I graduated from college with a degree in photography and, within several years, I'd established a successful career path as a media producer. After developing MS at 27, I lived with increasing disabilities over the years that followed and could no longer meet the physical demands of the work. I reinvented myself time and again, only to discover that I couldn't do what I thought I could because of ever-changing limitations.

Some people try to learn as much as possible about the course of their illness, only to discover huge variations occur in what can happen and when. Trying to predict your health based on statistics or what happened to your friend's neighbor's brother's cousin is probably as reliable as going to a fortune-teller. It takes determination to look at decreasing possibilities and refuse to crumble. It takes courage to face the loss of what you could do and see opportunity in its place.

When I turned 39, I decided I needed a major career change before my fortieth birthday. I'd lived with MS for 12 years, and I saw that it could affect how I worked for the rest of my life. I'd achieved a measure of success in my field, and I was committed to working because it gave me strength in the face of my physical weakness. It also gave me a sense of normalcy, in spite of my abnormal body. And I loved the act of working and its rewards. But I was married with two young children, and I recognized that working took a lot of my energy. I had to love what I was doing for it to be worth the effort.

I decided that what I wanted most was to go to law school. I had a vision of myself as an advocate for those who truly needed it. I thought I could do this, even if I ended up in a wheelchair. But illness intervened big time, and a few months short of my fortieth birthday, I was diagnosed with a second autoimmune disease, ulcerative colitis.

I became sicker than ever before, and I had to stop working altogether. Although I was still determined to continue to be productive and earn an income, it was difficult to imagine how I could even complete the law school coursework. It seemed even less likely that I could ever hold a job, with my health and at my age, in this competitive field.

As a compromise, I trained as a mediator—a career that involved hours, not years, of education. It turned out that I enjoyed this work more than I probably would have cared for practicing law.

Fortunately, a few years later, I had surgery to remove my colon and was cured of the ulcerative colitis. Within 1 year, I was running an urban high school mediation program. I loved it, but eventually the early hours and long days were still too difficult, since the MS had become more active. Leaving that job, I knew that I needed a more flexible work schedule than a school system could offer.

Suddenly, the solution seemed obvious: I would become self-employed.

It took 10 years to develop the skills and knowledge to be successful in my work. Even more important, each step had to be very thoughtful, because I had neither the strength nor the resources to waste. But I developed a plan, following it when I could and modifying it when I couldn't. I love what I do, and I recognize that it took a lot of determination to get here.

Obviously, careers can shift and turn in many ways—and no two journeys will be alike—but some common themes occur:

You want to change your job because AD symptoms make it difficult to do the work you were hired to do.

Rebecca is an x-ray lab technician, a job that requires manual dexterity and fine motor coordination. But due to the symptoms of scleroderma—tightening and stiffness in her hands—she's finding that she can no longer do the essential tasks of her job. She knows that she has to move on, and she's wondering how she can stay employed when she's trained to do only this job.

Obviously, when something like this happens, finding another job that requires the same tasks won't solve the problem. Therefore, you need to think about the issue within a larger context: how else and where else can you apply your talents?

This is when you must assess your skills and your competencies. Career counselors can be very valuable in helping you think creatively, so that you can leverage your capabilities and minimize your weaknesses.

Whatever you do, don't waste time fretting about the need to invest in the time and training required to take on a different a job. Don't put energy into worrying about whether or not you'll be able to perform this new job as you move down the road. Just keep in mind that there are no guarantees in life, and it's impossible to accurately predict the course of anyone's future— AD notwithstanding. The best you can do is make educated guesses based on what you know about your illness course thus far and the shape you're in now.

Although you can still do your job, you believe it's likely that at some point this won't be the case.

Karen is 42, with a master's degree in elementary education, and has been teaching first grade for 15 years. The symptoms from MS are making it increasingly difficult for her to stand on her feet all day. So far, she's found ways to compensate, but she worries that it's going to become more difficult as she gets older.

She dreams about changing careers, and has considered going into the business world to become a corporate trainer. On the other hand, she also thinks about going into education administration. Either way, she feels that these jobs won't require as much physical mobility, although she realizes that she'll need additional skills and training.

When circumstances such as this arise, it's a good time to speak with people who do the kind of work that

Ask Your Network:
- How do they think you should apply your talents?
- What do they know about your career ideas and the industries you're considering?
- Whom do they know that you might talk with to get more specific information?

you're considering. They can be a good source of information on the nature of the job market, specific career opportunities, and the effect your physical limitations might have on your job prospects. Use your network. Start by talking with friends and close colleagues to get their ideas, and ask the questions listed in the accompanying sidebar. When you pursue this kind of proactive planning, you're using your warrior skills.

You're looking for a new job, and you want to be sure that you've explored all the angles to ensure that it will be a good fit.

Recruiters advise employers to hire people for their competencies and overall fit with the organization, rather than focusing on specific experience and skills. As an employee who lives with AD, it's a wise idea to look carefully at a company's culture as well as job specifications.

The fact is that you're more likely to thrive in an organization that promotes employee-friendly policies. Over the long run, a broad range of benefits, employee development programs, and a flexible work policy can be more valuable than salary. Make sure you interview your potential supervisor concerning his or her values and support for people with differences.

◇◇◇◇◇◇◇◇◇◇◇◇◇◇◇◇◇◇◇◇◇◇◇◇◇◇◇◇◇◇◇◇◇◇◇◇◇◇

Evaluate If a Job Is Right for You— Whether You're Currently Employed or Shopping Around

If you're planning to stay in your job or field, ask yourself:

- Do I have the knowledge and skills to do this job well?
- If not, what do I need in terms of training and experience? Is it worth the expense to get it?
- Do I like what I do well enough to do it on both good days and bad?
- Can I do the job when my symptoms worsen?
- Is there room for me to grow?
- Is this something I want to do—and can plan to do—for the long run?
- Is there a market for my skills in other industries if the one I'm currently working in has a downturn?

If you're dealing with advancement issues, ask yourself:

- Is this job usually a stepping-stone to a higher position?

(continued)

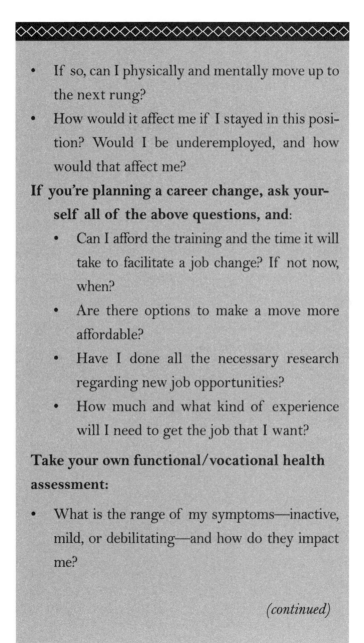

- If so, can I physically and mentally move up to the next rung?
- How would it affect me if I stayed in this position? Would I be underemployed, and how would that affect me?

If you're planning a career change, ask yourself all of the above questions, and:

- Can I afford the training and the time it will take to facilitate a job change? If not now, when?
- Are there options to make a move more affordable?
- Have I done all the necessary research regarding new job opportunities?
- How much and what kind of experience will I need to get the job that I want?

Take your own functional/vocational health assessment:

- What is the range of my symptoms—inactive, mild, or debilitating—and how do they impact me?

(continued)

- What are the skills, competencies, and physical/mental abilities required by my current job?
- Do the limitations posed by my symptoms allow me to meet these requirements?

Identify the best type of work environment for you:

- What matters most to me: work hours, commute, company philosophy, salary, benefits?
- Do I want the job for the long run (several years or more) or as a quick turnaround?
- Is there opportunity for growth, and will my illness play a role in my ability to move ahead?
- How much job flexibility do I need? Will it be available to me?
- What is the corporate culture like? Do the actions of the company support its philosophy? Are policies employee-friendly?
- Can I expect support from my boss?
- Can I realistically find everything I'm looking for? (This is a tough one, and you'll need to prioritize.)

According to research done by J.E. Beaty in her doctoral dissertation "Chronic Illness Disclosure in the Workplace," a supportive boss can make a dramatic difference regarding the ability of an employee with chronic illness to thrive at work (1).

Finally, take a good hard look at the financial health of the industry and the individual company. It's not in your best interest to change jobs frequently if you have disabling symptoms and need accommodations. It's far easier to get what you need when you're already a proven entity and people like and respect you. If jobs are in jeopardy due to market forces (such as production moving to other countries or shrinking demand), the overall culture will be demoralized, less flexible, and unable to offer you the long-term stability you need.

It can be difficult to leave a situation that you know and where you are known. It takes some compelling reasons to drive a person to look for a different job or a new career, and living with AD can be one such reason. By carefully considering why you are moving on, with as much honesty as you can muster, you can develop the fortitude to keep pushing when things get tough.

Keep this in mind: a warrior spirit includes well-developed plans, clear-sighted focus, and the ability to leap for what you want. When you're a warrior in balance, you have the strength and stability to face whatever comes your way.

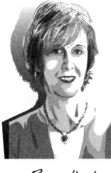

Rosalind

4

The Relationship Among Diagnosis, Disease Course, and Career Development

Most of us live our lives day to day, without serious periods of long-range planning. However, life-cycle experts take a more clinical approach by observing the bigger picture. Renowned psychologists, social scientists, and career researchers have developed models of life and career stages to identify and explain typical evolutionary phases.

Career Theory Models

In the world of career theory, which emerged as a field of study in the mid twentieth century, careers are thought of as the sequence of jobs people hold across time, incorporating an individual's evolving identity and social structures. Identity plays a central role in the vocation a person chooses and the way her career progresses.

As originally conceived, career models were based on chronological age, reflecting the normal and prevalent patterns of marriage, sexuality, and child-rearing. It was a linear pattern, with one step inevitably leading to the next.

But, over the past three decades, a dramatically different economy and workforce have altered the landscape. Following World War II, a blue- or white-collar worker in the United States could expect to be employed by a single organization for his entire work life. He could be confident that the company would take care of him—with good health benefits, sufficient training that would allow for advancement, and a job that would always be there. But this notion has been turned upside-down.

Let's start with the make-up of the workforce. Initially, career research focused on relatively young white men because...well, they're the ones who had careers. These days, the workforce is more multicultural, more female, and comprised of an increasingly older population. These individuals have needs that a previously homogeneous workforce did not.

In particular, the dramatic increase in the numbers of women in the workforce over the last half of the twentieth century is shaping what a career path looks like. Women face a particular set of challenges, unique to their gender, when they address their work lives. They tend to make decisions based on personal circumstances, and that creates a dynamic interaction between career and personal choices.

There's also the marketplace we call the New Economy. According to Frederick Reichheld in his book *The Loyalty Effect*, the fact that entire industries are moving to other continents and small businesses are being consumed by mega organizations means that employment is more fluid and less job loyalty exists (1). Where once predictable career stages existed, now a more dynamic experience is the norm. And perhaps what is most significant is the fact that individuals, instead of "the organization," are finding themselves responsible for developing the course of their careers.

In the early 1980s, Donald Super wrote an article entitled "A Life Span, Life-Space Approach to Career Development," which appeared in the *Journal of Vocational Behavior* (2). It described a five-stage model of career development that includes growth, exploration, establishment, maintenance, and disengagement. He suggested that levels of commitment to work roles vary over time. Priorities, obligations, and goals change in accordance with evolving family patterns and personal development, such that people will invest more or less of themselves in their work roles depending on other commitments.

For example, parents of young children may shift their focus to greater family involvement and less work involvement. The goals of late-career workers often shift to "generativity," as they focus on developing the next generation's skills and giving back to the community. The connections and trade-offs that occur between work and personal life figure prominently in recent career research.

Career and Autoimmune Disease

Living with autoimmune disease (AD) means that there is a third influence on your choices, because a chronic illness plays a strong role in the decisions you make in both your personal life and your career. The good news is that in this New Economy, women with AD can obtain jobs more easily than in previous decades. The sheer number of females in the workforce makes it easier to get jobs, because today's women don't face the barriers experienced by previous generations.

At the same time, recent advances in drug therapies and treatment for several ADs (as well as other chronic illnesses) have meant that more women living with AD can and do work. Although it is still not easy, the numbers make it more possible than ever to find a job that offers the flexibility you need to take care of your health, fulfill your personal life, and experience career growth.

This is all good news. But depending on where you are in your life or career stage, chronic illness can wreak havoc with your identity, and that strongly influences the choices you make.

When Joy was 15 years old, she developed Crohn's disease. She couldn't participate in team sports any longer, and she struggled to keep up in school. The disease left her worn and tired, and she spent weeks studying alone at home. She went from being an outgoing, bubbly girl to a quiet and shy young woman.

Although her four siblings went to college, Joy's parents supported her decision to drop out in her junior year. They didn't think she would need the degree, because they didn't think she'd be healthy enough to work.

When Joy married a few years later, she and her husband decided not to have children, because they'd heard that Crohn's could worsen during pregnancy. Joy took a job in a large manufacturing company near her home and, over the years, her bosses periodically encouraged her to earn a college degree so that she could get a promotion.

But Joy didn't think it made sense. She'd always seen herself as vulnerable, and she didn't like to take risks. She strongly believed that it was likely she'd get too sick to work if she took on more responsibility. In truth, she was relatively healthy and symptom-free for 20 years.

When her husband died suddenly when Joy was 48, she had to support herself. An experienced accounts-payable clerk, she realized that she was perfectly capable of doing so. This awareness made her life look very different.

She started swimming at the local indoor pool and, for the first time in her memory, she wanted to push harder. No longer afraid of what might happen, she didn't fear what might be ahead. She enrolled in community college to earn her degree, and applied at work for a highly specialized training program in technical sales that would give her the chance to travel and learn new skills.

For the first time since she was 15, Joy doesn't worry about maintaining her health at the cost of everything else. She has options, and she's glad for that.

Diagnosed as a teenager when she was developing her sense of self, Joy's identity formed around chronic illness. The knowledge of her affliction and her feeling of vulnerability became the basis on which she made her life decisions. While this allowed her to take her health into account, it also constricted her options.

Given the course of her illness, which improved over time, Joy became more convinced that not pushing herself physically would allow her to stay healthy. Most of all, she believed that this was critical to her happiness. But when she hit a life-transforming event—the loss of her husband—she experienced a shift in her attitude about work and her need to do whatever it took to maintain her health. Although this happened at a time in life when many people want to pull back from career and focus more on family and self, Joy's life and career had been limited, and she was ready for some expansion.

According to Robert Lahita's book, *Women and Autoimmune Disease,* an autoimmune disease in which onset is predominantly between the ages of 25 and 40—the prime childbearing and career-building years—inevitably interacts with a woman's career path by changing her abilities, priorities, and career goals (3). Where you are in your career and your life will always influence the decisions you make. And, while you don't have complete control of your health, you *do* have control over the way in which chronic illness influences your decision-making process.

In her senior year of college, after developing odd symptoms in her hands, Jessica was diagnosed with scleroderma. She knew a little about the disease, because her best friend's mom was disabled by it. At first she wasn't too concerned, because her symptoms were so slight. She knew better than to ignore them, however, because she had watched her friend's mom struggle so much over the years.

Jessica had been studying to teach elementary school, but thought such work would be too difficult if the disease progressed. Instead, she decided that it would be prudent to train as an accountant, thinking it was a small price to pay to be able to continue to work. When she graduated, she was fortunate enough to get a good entry-level job in a large accounting firm, where she was told she would be able to advance.

Soon she was making good money, better than she would have made as a teacher. But after 5 years, Jessica was bored and miserable. The disease hadn't become any worse, and she wasn't as worried about her future. She decided to go back to teaching and take her chances with her health.

Single and with few encumbrances, Jessica was able to move to another state where prospects for teaching jobs were better. It took a while to find employment since she had no experience, but she was willing to take a pay cut to get into the field. She feels it's more important to like what she does and to do it for as long as she can, rather than work at something she doesn't enjoy because it seems safe.

Let's look at the intersecting stages. Jessica was in an early stage of career development and life when she first developed her illness. Given her personal experience with the disease, her first instinct was to prioritize in favor of what she hoped would keep her healthy. She tried to adapt her career goals to what she thought would be her health needs. Because she'd been trained but hadn't devoted time to developing professional skills, and because she had no personal responsibilities, such as a family to support, it was relatively easy for her to make the shift to accounting. Switching back to teaching was more difficult, because she'd achieved some career stride in accounting, with a good pay scale and measurable success. But her youth and lack of personal responsibilities allowed her the flexibility to make the professional changes.

When Trudy was in graduate school in her early twenties, she became extremely tired. She was ultimately diagnosed with pernicious anemia, which improved with medication. Several years later, she noticed that she had droopy eyelids (ptosis), and thought it was due to long hours and stress at her job. When she became pregnant with her first child, her obstetrician noticed the problem and suggested that she see an eye doctor. Trudy hated going to doctors and ignored the advice, thinking her condition would improve after childbirth.

Not long after her child was born, she developed problems around her mouth that made it difficult to speak. Several specialists later, she was diagnosed with myasthenia gravis. The medication she was prescribed dramatically improved her fatigue and muscle weakness, and she was able to manage the disease over the years.

At the age of 45—while she was successfully running her own business as a biologist and her two children were in high school—Trudy began to experience the severe muscle weakness and eye droop again. As the major breadwinner in the family, she couldn't afford to leave her job. Nor did she want to.

The myasthenia gravis continued to worsen, and it became difficult for Trudy to run her business. She decided to try a new medication, but was warned that the side effects could be difficult. She realized that she'd have to make changes in her organization if she wanted to keep it afloat.

Trudy knew she was fortunate to have been able to build her career in the way she had. Although she felt that her strong track record would help keep her business running, she acknowledged that she'd have to hire more help and offload some responsibilities. She was willing to reduce her salary, if necessary, to keep from losing too much ground.

Trudy accomplished what she set out to do and, as she put it, "managed to tread water" over the next few years. By the time both her sons had graduated from college, her expenses had decreased and she could afford to cut back even further. Instead, she opted to expand her business, since her illness was no longer as active as it had been.

Let's take a look at another woman facing change in midlife:

Sandy is 50, single, and has three children. Before she was married, she taught high school science for 2 years and loved it, but always knew that she'd be a stay-at-home mom while her kids were young.

A few years ago, she had trouble walking and was diagnosed with rheumatoid arthritis. When she and her husband divorced a year later, she desperately needed to earn an income. She wanted to go back to teaching, but worried that she might not be able to continue if her physical problems got worse.

Sandy has opted to take a job as a classroom teacher for a few years to see how she will fare. She's also taking courses

*toward a master's degree in education administration, and
the school system is footing the bill. If the time comes when
she can no longer teach because of her physical limitations,
she hopes to find work as an administrator—a job that is
less physically demanding and also pays better.*

In these stories, the women described are making decisions based upon health, career, and personal
issues. To do this in your own life, you will need to
take stock of your personal goals.

Are you at the beginning or the end of your
career? Are you starting a family, are your kids grown,
or are you just getting into the dating pool? What
stage are you in regarding your AD? Are symptoms
easily managed, or are you in need of daily down-
time and doctor visits? Are you angry and depressed
to the point where you aren't functioning well in
your relationships with others? Are you feeling such
grief that you can't imagine hope or happiness ever
again?

All of these factors play into each other. Your ability to look at each one and understand how it influences the others will allow you to make decisions that
give you the flexibility and hope you need.

Stages of Chronic Illness

Looking at chronic illness as a life event that takes place in evolving and resolving stages allows you to see where you are and what might be ahead. From my work and discussions with women who have AD, I've identified stages of illness that are similar to personal and career stages. Let's take a look.

Diagnosis

For most people, symptoms lead to a diagnosis. But others can have symptoms for years before knowing what the problem is—and some are never diagnosed at all. Having a diagnosis can be a real turning point in how you view your illness. It can be a tremendous relief, particularly if you have spent considerable time and energy hunting for an explanation. A diagnosis gives you confirmation that your symptoms are "real" and you actually fit into a category. This is a time when many women try to learn about the disease and find a doctor who can help with treatment.

When Molly was in college, she had frequent stomach aches and what she called "bathroom problems." Her family internist recommended various over-the-counter drugs and told her to avoid stress. Sometimes the medicine seemed to help. But avoid stress? She was in college!

A few years later, when she was working in her first job, Molly's bowel problems became increasingly frequent and demanding. Her doctor gave her a prescription medication, but it didn't help. A year later, 6 years after the onset of her stomach problems, Molly saw blood in her stool. She became terrified that she was dying. Her doctor sent her to a gastroenterologist and, after blood tests and a colonoscopy, she was diagnosed with ulcerative colitis (UC). Molly knew nothing about UC, but was relieved it wasn't cancer. How bad could this be?

Denial

Many women experience a period following diagnosis when they forget—or try to forget—that illness is a factor in their lives. This is difficult to do when you're struggling with extreme symptoms, but when the illness is quiet, it's easy to convince yourself that there's been a mistake. Better yet, maybe you're one of the lucky ones who gets miraculously better.

Some people find themselves making bargains: *If I get enough sleep, I won't get sicker.* Others wonder if there was a misdiagnosis: *Maybe I'm really not sick after all.* Still others opt to minimize the entire issue: *I've been symptom-free for 2 weeks, so it's not that big a deal.* While denial is not a negative emotion in and of itself, it becomes harmful when you ignore an issue that is real and requires your attention. The positive side of denial is that it can serve as a tool that allows you to keep living your life without being paralyzed by fear.

Molly's first big flare of UC calmed down within several weeks with medication. At the advice of her mom's friend who had UC, she briefly looked into various diets that might help her stay healthy. She soon lost interest in the plan, and told herself she just wanted to return to life as she'd known it. She stayed on the medication, and experienced only occasional and mild problems.

A few years later, when she and her boyfriend started talking about marriage, she realized that her denial of her condition had prevented her from telling him about it. She finally shared the information, and he countered with the fact that his aunt had UC, and it had been difficult for her to have children. Molly angrily responded that it wasn't a problem, because she didn't have the disease anymore.

This was a period of intense career development for Molly, who was on the fast track at the investment firm where she worked, and was also taking courses for her MBA. When she was offered a job that required a lot of travel, she decided the timing was great. Although marriage plans were in the works, she and her fiancé didn't intend to have children for a few years. Molly briefly weighed the idea of discussing the UC with her mentor, an older woman who had been very helpful in her career choices. She ultimately decided against it, since she believed that the illness really wasn't a factor in her life.

Anger

After the relief of diagnosis and the quiet of denial, anger can set in when symptoms flare or the disease progresses. The possibility of ongoing disabilities becomes real, and you get just plain mad.

You feel furious with your doctor: *Why can't you find a treatment that makes me feel better?* You're fuming at your spouse, partner, or best friend: *Why can't you understand what I need?* And you're livid with your boss: *Why can't you support me?*

Then there's the flip side of anger—depression— and it's always focused on you: *My life is horrible, and it's all my fault.* Some women swing back and forth between denial and anger/depression, particularly if their symptoms wax and wane.

Molly loved her position, and didn't mind the travel. Her new husband worked long hours, and they were sav- ing money so they could eventually buy a house when they were ready to start a family. After almost a year into the new job, Molly developed very severe UC symptoms. Her doctor put her on an aggressive medication and, although the symptoms improved somewhat, the side effects of the medication left her weak, tired, and unable to maintain her busy schedule.

She found herself snapping at everyone around her and, although she didn't tell anyone at work that she was sick, she felt deeply frustrated that others weren't more supportive. Suddenly she resented the stress of her job. She was furious with her husband for even mentioning that they should start a family—and he wouldn't even do the laundry! Her friends didn't understand when she told them how she felt or when she'd break the plans they had made.

The flare subsided after 6 months, but it was only a temporary reprieve. Molly's symptoms would get worse, without any rhyme or reason, every few months—sometimes lasting for just a few days. She started to withdraw from everyone around her and just wanted to stay in bed.

Molly was angry. How could this happen? How could she plan her career or a family? She blamed her doctor for not being more aggressive with her disease earlier on, and for failing to tell her it could get so bad. She was furious with her boss for not understanding when she needed time off. And she felt that her husband was letting her down by not picking up the slack at home and taking better care of her.

Grief

According to grief expert Elisabeth Kübler-Ross, there are five stages of grieving. For the sake of simplicity, we're going to view them as one.

Grief is an emotion that is often overlooked when talking about chronic illness, but it is critical to any discussion about living with AD—which translates into learning to live with loss. That's not to say that there aren't gains here, too. But loss is inevitable, even at the basic level of not being able to do or feel as you once did.

But unlike a death, this loss isn't final. Instead, you're struggling to come to terms with losing something that is changing: *Yesterday I couldn't lift my leg, today I can, and I'm not sure about tomorrow.* The change can be gradual and take place over time: *I finally realize that I need to use the bathroom every 2 hours.* It is often unnoticed until you discover that you can no longer do something you once could: *When I dropped the bowl, I knew I couldn't use that hand to grab things.* We grieve not only for what our bodies no longer can do, but for the loss of our sense of who we are.

If the loss becomes more permanent, and you have time to live with it and adapt, you might find that you're not angry or depressed anymore. Instead, you feel sad. You find yourself moving back and forth between anger and grief, but at some point you experience grief without anger.

Over the next few years, Molly struggled with symptoms that never seemed to go away for long. In her early thirties, she worried about putting off pregnancy, but she and her husband adhered to their commitment not to have children at this time. Her health didn't seem very stable, and she would have to go off medication if she became pregnant. She also knew that her firm wouldn't allow her to work a flex schedule until she'd moved up the career ladder, so she wanted to give herself a few more years of working before making a change. She also realized that she was too consumed with her own loss over this illness to be able to be a good parent.

Molly knew that she was severely depressed when she couldn't shake her sadness and disappointment, so she sought professional help. It enabled her to view herself differently and to make more time for herself without feeling guilty. She took yoga classes to strengthen and relax her body, and made more of an effort to enjoy being with her husband, family, and friends.

Acceptance

One day, out of the blue, you wake up and discover that you can't do something you could do just yesterday. Instead of getting deeply upset, you simply make the necessary course correction and move on. This, girl-friend, is the acceptance phase.

You realize you've experienced loss, but if you've been fortunate enough to grow in each stage up to this point, you're aware that there have been gains from your increasing knowledge about yourself. Acceptance doesn't mean having no regrets when you want to do something but can't. It means recognizing the feelings and thoughts for what they are, and not allowing them to control you.

On her thirty-fifth birthday, Molly decided that she had to get on with her life plans and decided to try to get pregnant. She went off her medication and, within a few months, she conceived. Her pregnancy had some rough spots, but she was able to continue to work through most of it. Before she went on maternity leave, she disclosed her illness to her boss (she was now a director), and discussed the option of taking unpaid time off for a few months after the baby was born if she wasn't well. She also talked about reducing her hours on a trial basis. Molly felt confident that this was the best she could do for now.

You'll recognize the acceptance stage as soon as you reach it. And it might even make you smile.

When our daughters were in college, my husband and I wanted to take a family vacation that we'd all enjoy. We chose Costa Rica, because it would have beaches (for the girls), physical challenges (for my husband), and beautiful outdoors (for me). I had no idea what I was getting into.

Over the previous 5 years, I'd grown healthier than I'd been since my first diagnosis, but I still hesitated to take physical risks, given my history. On the other hand, I didn't like to make a show of this to our daughters, always wanting them to see me as upbeat and strong about my health.

For the first 15 years of living with MS, I chose to ignore my disabilities. Whenever I could, I pushed myself to be like everyone else. I ended up with broken legs and arms and lots of mishaps. As time went by, I became more afraid and less willing to challenge myself physically, simply because life felt like challenge enough.

When we planned the Costa Rica trip, we didn't even consider my health to be a factor, as we might have 5 years prior, when I was much more disabled. As a result, we didn't realize that the sights we wanted to see required arduous hikes down steep ravines and horseback rides that guaranteed leg bruises. After the first experience, in which I had to slide down a muddy mountain because my balance was so bad, I felt furious with myself for agreeing to this vacation without researching it more carefully. I hated that my daughter had to slow her pace to stay with me. I felt depressed that, once again, I was limited.

That night, I was miserable at dinner and wouldn't talk to my family. I had grown daughters who read my signals and although I wanted to be an adult, I felt and acted like a child. I was disappointed that, after all these years, I was still letting my disabilities get me down. As I struggled to pull myself together—telling myself that being angry about what I couldn't change was not a grown-up response—I had an epiphany.

I realized that, although I'd thought I had accepted my life with my physical limitations, it wasn't completely true. When challenged by something new or in a different setting, I wasn't fully integrating my new self. The next day, I gratefully took my daughter's hand as we traversed a mild waterfall. And when I slipped and fell and my husband had to lift me because I couldn't get my balance, I wasn't upset. I actually felt glad that I was able to do what I couldn't have done several years earlier. The following day, I chose not to go on a hike and stayed by the pool instead. I was glowing with happiness just to be there.

Throughout your life, three factors—health, career, and personal issues—continuously intersect as they shift in their level of priority. Your response to your illness will be influenced by the career and personal events that take place.

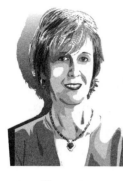

Rosalind

5

Success in the Workplace: When Knowledge and Experience Are Not Enough

Over the past decade, a subtle yet dramatic shift has occurred in the workplace. The 40-hour work-week, long considered the gold standard, has quietly and insidiously stretched into 50 to 60 hours. Despite this accepted practice, social commentators and the average person agree that functioning at such a pace can't possibly be good for one's mental or physical health.

So I ask you: if the expanded work-week isn't healthy for someone in good physical condition, how can it possibly be acceptable for someone with a chronic illness? Quite simply, it's not.

When you live with autoimmune disease (AD), you can't afford to push yourself in such a manner. If, by some bizarre quirk, you're managing to do it, odds are it's a serious struggle. Sadly, too many people with chronic illness berate themselves or feel inadequate because they can't "keep up." If you're working in a high-paced, frenetic, multitasking environment, and you live with an AD that slows you down, it's easy to feel distressed by your cognitive or physical impairment. It's also easy to lose sight of the alternatives at your disposal and to view not working at all as your only option.

In truth, it really is possible to stay successfully employed. It might require taking a different job with fewer responsibilities. It might mean enduring a drop in salary. It almost certainly necessitates developing a radically different approach to *how* you work. The bottom line is that you need to be able to choose when and how to walk rather than run. And this requires developing the competence to think, plan, and act strategically to stay in the workplace.

So, strap on your warrior suit and take on the challenge. It won't be easy…it will take a noble effort… but the opportunity to take charge of your life is well worth it.

When Meredith was a junior in college, she developed frequent fevers, then a rash, and finally anemia. Her doctor diagnosed her with lupus, put her on drug therapy, and told her to take off the rest of the semester. Delighted when she quickly went into remission, she returned to school and went on to earn a master's degree in public health, hoping to work in public policy in Third World countries. Upon graduating, she took a job that seemed to be a perfect fit for her training, and she was excited by the frequent travel and high performance goals. She loved the work and the autonomy.

After 1 year on the job, the lupus returned. The fevers left Meredith feeling exhausted, and her swollen joints made it hard to get around. Her solo position meant that the work didn't get done unless she did it and, over the next year, for the first time in her life, she felt that she was underperforming.

She stayed on for another year, hoping the disease would settle down again. But when her boss suggested that she might not be well-suited to the job's fast pace and pressure, she jumped at a friend's suggestion to leave and go to work in his small consulting group.

Meredith thought this new opportunity would give her the chance to slow down and regain her health. However, the symptoms didn't improve, and her physical condition seemed to be more of a problem than ever. Caught in the throes of a project-driven environment—where everyone pitched in and relied on each other heavily—she was always struggling or letting someone down. To compound the situation, the company offered limited healthcare benefits, which posed a serious problem for Meredith.

Miserable, she thought about stopping work altogether, but her financial situation would not allow it. Instead, she took a job with a large healthcare organization that espoused an employee-friendly culture and featured great health benefits. Although her new role was a step down in job responsibility, she was committed to seeing it through.

She worked first on a team with a strong cooperative spirit, which was an unusual and difficult role after having worked so extensively on her own. Persistence and tenacity paid off, and she eventually became the team leader. Although this is by no means her dream job, it has taught her the value of working in an environment that allows her to succeed in spite of her unpredictable health.

Too many people who live with chronic illness describe their lives as "fighting a war," and each day feels like a battle. The ability to accomplish day-to-day tasks can suddenly change as symptoms wax and wane, frequently and unpredictably. Even if you're willing to push your limits and risk wearing yourself down, you might worry that disabling symptoms will prevent you from leading a satisfying and fruitful life. You might be afraid or hesitant to acknowledge what you need, but if you allow yourself to slip into denial, it can lead you to ignore your experiences and mounting difficulties.

Does it make sense to do double duty just to prove that you can? If you're already running on empty when you shift into first gear, working only increases the strain. But that doesn't mean you have to stop altogether. An alternative is to develop your capacity to think strategically about work and develop the competence you need to achieve your desired outcomes.

So, what exactly does that look like?

Recognize what you want and need.

Identify what matters to you at the moment, instead of continuing to do what you've always done or what you think you should do. For example: *Even though I'm trained and experienced in elementary education, I don't have the physical energy to stand all day in a classroom. I want to keep working, but I need to do something less physically demanding.*

Establish your desired outcomes.

Decide where you want to be, or what you want to achieve. For example: *I want to figure out what kind of job I can get that allows me to use my background and expertise, affords the flexibility I need when I'm not feeling well, and allows me to continue to be successful.*

Create a plan for action and develop new competencies.

Map out the direction in which you want to move, and determine the skills you'll need to get there. For example: *I will research the training field on the Internet, and speak with several people I know who are trainers. I'll find out what jobs I might be suited for, develop a résumé, and network to find what positions are available. I need to learn how to do this kind of research, how to tailor my résumé, and how to interview in a competitive market. I need to be able to make good decisions about the kind of job I can perform well and the type of environment I prefer.*

I don't want to give the impression that this will be a straightforward experience. It rarely is. My journey to discover the values of setting a goal and thinking strategically had twists, bumps, and even craters in the road.

At the time when I was diagnosed with MS, I was looking forward to progressing to my dream job: that of a multimedia producer. Such jobs require frequent travel, late nights, tight deadlines, and lots of physical energy—all of which I craved. But now I was faced with the prospect of being bedridden for weeks, losing my vision, or not being able to walk. Everything I heard about this illness made it clear that the work schedule of a producer could prove particularly difficult—and might even make me sicker. For the first time in my life, health factors came into play when determining a career move, and they would continue to affect my decisions as time went on.

Ten years, two children, and four jobs later, I was teaching communications at a university with one thought in mind: teaching college is something I can do no matter how bad the MS symptoms get, so I'm going to keep at it. But when I developed ulcerative colitis, another AD disease, I had a far more difficult set of disabilities: demanding bathroom issues, high fevers, and sapped energy.

There's no backup when you teach college, so I dragged my sorry body to work each day, barely making it through my classes. And then I experienced another first: poor performance reviews. One year later, I stopped working—ostensibly to get my health under control, but also because I was too tired to keep going.

When I was diagnosed with MS, my neurologist, seeing how distressed I was, took my hand and said, "Rosalind, you're too young to understand this, but illness can be an opportunity. It can teach you to see clearly what really matters to you."

It was only when I left that job that I realized why being part of the workforce was so important to me.

It allowed me to feel normal, even in the face of my abnormal health. It gave me a sense of competence—in my skills and my ability to earn a living—that I desperately needed, regardless of pain or fatigue.

But I also recognized that I needed a plan. I couldn't just take the first opportunity that came along or take a job because it appealed to me, as I'd always done. So, I set a long-term goal: to have a job that wouldn't leave me vulnerable to my unpredictable health. I needed to have flexibility with scheduling. I didn't want to put a lot of money and time into getting more education or training, since I wasn't convinced my plan would work. I'd have to love what I was doing, or I wouldn't have the energy to do it. And finally, I'd need a lot of patience, because I had no idea how long it would take to implement my plan. As it turned out, carving my own path at my own speed allowed me the opportunity for real success. It took 10 years, but I'm here.

Having a goal gave me something to work toward and to measure against. I determined the worth of any activity against a single standard: will this help me achieve my goal? If not, I eliminated it. Strategic thinking allowed me to move from focusing solely on immediate concerns and to invest in a long-term plan.

It's important to develop your resilience so that you can respond with your warrior spirit (*I can get up and do battle another day*) when careful planning doesn't work out as you'd intended.

With thoughtful strategies, you can be mentally prepared to meet what might arise, but you must also hone your skills and tactics. Your toolbox should include the expertise you already have and that which you need to acquire.

Developing Your Competence

Build a Team

When you work in an organization, you inevitably interface with others—either because you're part of a functional team, or because you are responsible to and/or for others. When you have the unpredictable factor of AD symptoms, the ideal solution is to be part of a team that has had a high degree of cross-training, so that if you have to step back or out for a period of time, the outcomes will not be affected.

Unfortunately, many organizations do not support cross-training. What's more, staffing might be such that the individuals with whom you work do not

Evaluating Symptoms That Could Get "In the Way" of Doing What Is "Expected" of You

Ask Yourself:

- What is different from my baseline experience ?

- How specifically does this change affect me ?

- How does this affect my ability to do my job?

- Can I overlook these symptoms and still get the job done?

- If I do overlook the symptoms, how will this impact how I feel, now and in the near future?

- If I don't do what is "expected" of me, will I feel better?

share your competencies. That's when it becomes your problem, and you have to wrestle with it until it's no longer a stumbling block.

Equally difficult is a situation in which you're the only one who can do your job—and if you can't do it, it doesn't get done. If symptoms prevent you from performing effectively and meeting deadlines, this is a tough position to sustain. Use the questions in the sidebar to help evaluate the situation.

Often, this kind of problem-solving involves managing up: effectively managing those who manage you so they're willing to lend their support or finance the accommodations or changes you suggest. This can be particularly difficult for some people, and it requires developing new competencies. But it's more than worth your effort, because it will increase your ability to influence others and provide important opportunities that you might otherwise miss.

Establish Allies and Advocates

Helen works as a nurse manager, with 12 people reporting directly to her. She has suffered from the periodic pain and fatigue of rheumatoid arthritis for the past 3 years, but her staff knows nothing about it. Helen fears that revealing her condition might jeopardize her career, yet her silence increasingly leaves her feeling lonely. In addition, she finds that she resents people who don't recognize what she accomplishes in spite of her difficulties—even though they're unaware of them. Helen considered quitting or taking a position with less responsibility and decided to talk with Cindy, a former boss, about the situation.

Cindy admitted that she'd noticed the changes in Helen over the past few years. Once very sociable with several good friends in the workplace, Cindy thinks that Helen has become withdrawn and somewhat aloof. While Cindy understands Helen's fears, she thinks Helen is hurting herself by her behavior. Since she's still performing her duties competently, Cindy suggested that Helen reach out to others before making a dramatic change, sharing her condition with a few old friends on staff and talking to her current boss about possible changes that might help.

Helen followed Cindy's advice. She found that one friend responded with a blank stare and never referred to it again. But the other two friends with whom she discussed her situation were warm and compassionate, inviting her to share more whenever she wants. When Helen spoke with her boss about the illness, her boss responded that she had been increasingly worried about Helen because she seemed remote and abrupt. She'd thought that Helen was burned out. Over their next two meetings, they were able to discuss what kinds of accommodations would support Helen and allow her to stay in her position while taking care of her health.

Helen made it clear that she didn't want others to know about her condition and she wasn't asking for major changes—only more flexibility in her scheduling. Her boss told her that it's difficult to find people with her experience and talents, and assured Helen that she would do anything possible to support her.

It's not always easy to open up to others, but it's better than feeling isolated. Sometimes, it can lead to substantial improvement in the workplace.

I've heard friends, colleagues, and clients say that living with chronic illness can be a lonely experience. You're surrounded by people who don't face the same challenges you do, and that makes you feel separate and different. You can't get any empathy or support if others don't know what you're going through. But sometimes, disclosing your condition to everyone at work isn't always a good idea.

So, what's a girl to do? Build allies and find advocates. Don't try to brave the storm alone, because it's tough enough dealing with work challenges. It's even harder when you're confronted with the difficult and unpredictable issues that arise from a chronic illness.

Allies are your friends, the people in whom you can confide and from whom you can get realistic feedback. For instance, if you're not sure whether your recent bad health has been a problem for others, or if you should take the job upgrade you've been offered, a trusted ally is someone who can help you figure things out. You need only one or two, and it's usually best if you choose people who don't work directly with you. Those who are removed from the immediate situation are in a better position to provide a neutral and honest assessment.

Advocates are the people who will go to bat for you. They might be supervisors, colleagues, or even support people. The key element they have in common is that they are aware of your strengths and talents, and are willing and able to speak up for you whenever necessary.

It's easy to see that everyone—perfectly healthy or not—would benefit from having allies and advocates at work. But they become even more valuable assets when you're faced with the challenges of chronic illness.

Simplify Decision-Making

Making a decision is easy when you have a clear preference for one option over another. But when the rhythm of your life is frequently upset by unpredictable health, good choices can be replaced by unpleasant alternatives.

Trying to make a decision based on your health can feel like wading into quicksand. And if you can't weigh your options relatively quickly, you could sink in that quicksand just trying to survive in the workplace.

Paula recognized the increasingly difficult symptoms she was experiencing from polymyalgia rheumatica (PMR) because she'd had them before. As the director of new product development for a software company, she was responsible for a large department and managed a sizeable budget. The timing couldn't have been worse, since her division was in the midst of its busiest season. She was faced with long workdays, frequent evening meetings, and the pressure of getting reports out in record time.

On days when she considered not going into work and staying home to rest, she inevitably opted to push herself because she didn't feel clear enough about how sick she really was. She had made an appointment to see her doctor, but canceled it at the last minute. Now, she faced a big decision.

Six months earlier, she had agreed to participate in a 3-day company off-site, thinking she could manage it because it would occur just as the busy season ended. With the off-site only 1 week away, she thought about not going. Again she hesitated, because she still couldn't tell how sick she was. She kept hoping the symptoms would get better, and she put off making a decision. When Paula finally decided not to go to the off-site, she was in the hospital.

Obviously, there isn't a universal response to these situations. Anyone with a chronic illness knows that activities that are possible under some circumstances can be unmanageable at other times. But you can manage the unpredictable with a mental model that helps you focus and eases the decision-making process. See the sidebar for some tips.

This isn't rocket science. But, in my experience, living with chronic illness can make high-achieving people dysfunctional. Fear—that we're going to make ourselves sicker if we keep going, that others will judge us poorly, or that we'll disappoint ourselves if we stop—can be a major stumbling block. It wastes precious resources, prevents us from moving at all, and could even make us unnecessarily sicker.

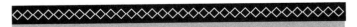

When you need to evaluate if and how to get the job done.

Ask Yourself:

- Are there creative approaches that I can tap into to do the job differently when I'm symptomatic?
- Can I get the necessary backup by sharing my job, even if it means less autonomy or less money?
- Can I get a different kind of support from those who work for me?

When making a decision in response to chronic illness symptoms, it is important to proceed just as you would when faced with any other business decision, big or small. By having a system in place, you take the emotion out of the equation and eliminate at least one stressor. And remember not to beat yourself up if you decide to go home instead of attending that meeting—only to find that you're feeling better before you even reach your front door. Maximize the time by using it to regenerate.

When You Can't Do What's Expected, Offer an Explanation

As a young person, I remember being struck by the truth of the expression "actions speak louder than words." As I've grown older, I've really come to appreciate the sheer power of words.

Consider this: how often do you find that, because of AD symptoms, your actions don't seem to support what you want to be doing? For instance, you want to get that report finished and distributed by this afternoon, but your intense fatigue makes it impossible to do anything. Sometimes, words are all you have to communicate your body's inaction.

But perhaps you're afraid to say you can't do something due to poor health because you think it will sound like an excuse. The word "excuse" has come to have a negative meaning—implying that you're hiding something or slacking off—when, in fact, an excuse is nothing more than an explanation, a reason. When you make it clear why you can't get a particular job done, you're not leaving it up to others to figure out what the problem is. You also avoid the possibility that they will fill in the blank with their own explanation, such as your incompetence or lack of motivation. However, there are times when saying "I'm sorry, I can't do it" isn't enough. You have to carefully consider what you say—and what you don't say.

Imagine that your boss wants you to take on a new project, but you're worried about agreeing to it because the scleroderma is flaring, and your hands have become too numb to use a keyboard. At a minimum, you should explain how the symptoms are affecting you and what you intend to do about it. You might name the disease or not, depending on whether it helps to clarify the situation.

Here are three things to keep in mind:

- Explain the problem that you are having in terms that another person can understand.
- Make it clear that you recognize the importance of the work.

- Demonstrate your commitment by offering a viable solution.

One response might be, "I'm sorry, but I can't do the project in the way that we discussed. My hands sometimes become numb from a chronic condition, and that causes trouble for me on the computer. I realize that it must be done by the end of the day today, so I'll get (someone else) on the team to do that part of the job while I handle the fieldwork."

When You Fail to Meet Expectations, Apologize

Everyone finds that there are times when it's impossible to meet expectations—both your own and those imposed by others. When you live with AD, this can be a frequent experience.

Do you find yourself thinking: *It's hard enough to let someone down, but I hate talking about it. It feels like I'm just rationalizing what I can't do.*

Or: *I can't tell anyone why I can't do this. My fatigue (pain, stiff limbs, you name it) just doesn't seem like a good enough excuse for not getting the work done.*

According to Aaron Lazare in his book, *On Apology,* an apology that includes why you are sorry and addresses the other person's concerns is the first step toward easing another's disappointment or anger with your actions (1). With an apology, you accept responsibility.

However, there are times when an apology is not enough, because the other party needs to know whether or not you can be relied upon in the future.

When All Else Fails, Fix the Problem

After you've given an explanation and offered an apology, the third step is to fix it so that it won't be repeated.

Fran works as a technical writer and lives with Sjögren's syndrome. She recently developed breathing problems, and found herself lightheaded and unfocused at work. When she realized that she had forgotten to include some documents in a report that a colleague needed, she was very upset. She was having a particularly bad day, and her mind felt like it was in a fog—something that had been happening with greater frequency.

She immediately apologized to her colleague, explaining that she wasn't feeling well and that her brain wasn't working properly. He knows that she has Sjögren's syndrome, and claims that he wants to be supportive. Under the circumstances, Fran thought he would be understanding, but that wasn't the case.

Instead, he brushed her off impatiently, saying "sorry" wasn't good enough and telling her he was getting tired of her mistakes. Fran was angry, deeply resentful of the fact that he didn't seem to comprehend how difficult work could be for her at times like this.

Fran's resentment toward her colleague's response is getting in the way of addressing a problem that is not going to disappear. She must ask herself if it's truly possible to perform her duties effectively and productively. The bottom line is painfully clear: if you can't do your job, you'll eventually be leaving it, because you'll either be fired or demoted.

If Fran believes that she can perform the functions of her job, she must develop solutions that support her. She might create back-up systems so that she can deliver even when her brain is fuzzy. She could delegate parts of her job to a co-worker or subordinate who is willing to take them on—even if it means that she loses some of her responsibilities, status, or power.

When you take on a job, any job, you must be able to perform reliably in order to be successful—chronic illness or not. An apology and an explanation will likely work when the incident is a one-time occurrence, but when the problem is a recurring one, you must be able to fix it. Otherwise, you lose your credibility, your support, and, ultimately, your job.

How Do You Know When Enough Is Enough?

In the 2004 playoffs against the New York Yankees, Boston Red Sox pitcher Curt Schilling injured his ankle. In spite of the problem, he decided to pitch the next game because he thought the team needed him. The Red Sox lost, and everyone was unhappy with his performance.

In the following game, however, his pitching improved and the Red Sox won. When the team went on to play in the World Series, Schilling's ankle was worse—visibly bleeding from temporary repair surgery—but he pitched brilliantly and the Red Sox famously won the World Series.

According to Schilling's own account, he couldn't walk on the morning he was to pitch in the World Series. He was certain he wouldn't/couldn't pitch that night. He later told reporters that when driving to work that morning, he saw road signs cheering him to win. His teammates hugged him when he arrived at the stadium. But in spite of this show of support... in spite of the fact that he had a multimillion-dollar contract to help the Boston Red Sox win the World Series... he told his manager he couldn't play.

Yet, that night, he was on the pitcher's mound. What happened? Did he overestimate his injury? Was his motiva-

tion so strong that he could ignore the pain and the possibility of further injury? And, if he could do that, what does that say about those of us who can't or choose not to?

When you live with a chronic illness, you often wonder how far you should push yourself. If you back away from a task, you worry that others will think you're "wimping out." After, all you *should* be able to do it. You could do it yesterday.

We think of chronic illness as being unpredictable, but chronic good health can be uncertain, as well. As in Schilling's case, you can't assume that you will always be able to deliver a peak performance. In fact, athletes regularly face the inevitability of injury so that they can respond appropriately should it happen. The truth is that no one knows what's around the corner, but living with chronic illness means that unpredictable health is more likely.

Sarah, a university professor, lives with Graves' disease and depression. She was halfway through the college semester, her health deteriorating rapidly, when her physician recommended a 1-week stay in the hospital. He told her that if she didn't take his advice, it was unlikely that she would be able to finish the semester.

Sarah was convinced she couldn't follow her doctor's

advice, fearing that her colleagues, who knew about her illness, would resent the fact that she was taking a leave in the middle of the semester. Her department chairperson would be angry that the burden might fall on him. And her students would be upset if she were to become unavailable.

When I asked her what would happen if she couldn't finish the semester, she said, "It would probably lead to losing this job—not now, but eventually."

After exploring her options, Sarah realized she could get coverage for her classes and responsibilities for the week, yet she was still reluctant to commit to the hospitalization and the time off. Even with extensive health constraints, she had always pushed herself, often to the brink of physical and mental exhaustion. She believed that was the reason she still had her job, and it took a brave leap of faith for her to commit to doing things differently.

Sarah decided to take a long weekend for the hospitalization, which meant she had to cancel only two classes. She developed materials for her teaching assistant to give to her students while she was in the hospital. She decided to inform her department chairman, because she knew he'd be very upset if he learned about this from another source. Sarah was able to assure him that her absence would not be a problem and would, in fact, allow her to successfully perform her duties for the remainder of the semester.

Sarah's chair never commented on her absence, nor did anyone else.

Curt Schilling probably always knew he'd be on the pitcher's mound that evening. His drive had brought him to this pinnacle and it would keep him going, because this was the World Series, and nothing would hold him back.

When we live with chronic illness, we can't possibly play as if every day is the World Series. There comes a time when you think, *It sure isn't working the way I'm doing it.* Today is always the right time to say, *enough is enough.*

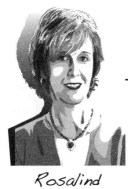

Rosalind

6

Talking About Your Chronic Illness

For many, the emotional challenges of living with an autoimmune disease (AD) are as significant as the physical ones. Some people are fortunate enough to get solace and support from their co-workers, but for others, work becomes a battleground of daily skirmishes pitting health against job. Stop for a moment, and ask yourself how things might be different if you were to talk openly about living with an AD.

Would disclosure improve your performance outcomes?

Is there a possibility that it might it be easier to change the way you work—such as slowing down, avoiding multitasking, finding alternative methods to get the job done—if others knew about your illness? Are specific accommodations available that would allow you to work better with disabling symptoms?

Would disclosure improve your chances for success?

If disabling symptoms are negatively impacting either the quantity or quality of what you deliver, people could be making incorrect assumptions about why this is happening. Would you get the support you need to be successful if others knew what you are up against?

If your answer to either question is that nothing would change, you probably don't need to read this chapter. There really is no reason to disclose your health status if doing so would not affect your performance or your ability to succeed.

The unfortunate truth is that disclosing an illness can be problematic. It usually means that you will have to confront other people's preconceptions and even their prejudices. You might also face their fear that you won't be able to do your job, or that your illness could become a costly burden. It's a sad reality that many organizations—and individuals, to boot—are not supportive of another's specific needs, no matter what they might claim.

Despite this fact, I believe that you're better off disclosing the situation if your condition impacts your ability to perform your job activities—or if you worry that they could. If this is the case, read on. You'll discover that, although there is hardly a one-size-fits-all solution to this complex issue, you can craft a strategy for how you conduct yourself at work. Furthermore, you can develop the competencies that allow you to implement that strategy.

To Disclose or not to Disclose—That is the Question

To disclose, according to the Merriam-Webster online dictionary, means to expose, to view, to make known or public. In this case, we're revealing information about ourselves that many consider to be private, even intimate, and certainly leaves us feeling vulnerable. Many of us share bits of who we are all the time—on matters both large and small—but when the information is as problematic as illness, it deserves very careful thinking.

Let's start with the caveat that when it comes to disclosing a chronic illness in the workplace, there isn't a right or wrong way to proceed. Because of the many variables of AD, it's nearly impossible to make a definitive statement about this complex issue.

Some people believe that you should never reveal a chronic illness in the workplace because of the bias surrounding it. We've all heard the stories—true or not—about the woman who was fired after disclosing her health problems, or never hired in the first place because she opted to be completely honest. Then there's the commonly held notion that others will think less of you if they know you have an illness. That can be true, but the fact remains that attitude about illness is changing.

As Baby Boomers age, all kinds of illness are more prevalent. Additionally, improved treatments are allowing people with AD to remain active and lead fairly normal lives. It's hard to find an organization—whether employing a staff of 10 or 200—that doesn't have at least one person who lives with an illness or debilitating condition of some sort. You're not as alone as you might think.

The decision whether or not to talk about your AD, however, does pop up primarily in three situations:

- During a job interview
- When you're already employed
- In ongoing communication with people who already know

Choosing to Disclose During a Job Interview

Melanie was diagnosed with diabetes when she was pregnant. She and her husband recently relocated, and she discovered that job opportunities in her field were slim. She began interviewing for a senior management position with a large manufacturing company, and she wanted the job very much. She'd held a similar position in her last job and is highly qualified. After several interviews for the new position, Melanie was told that she's a good fit. Her next meeting was scheduled with the person to whom she would report directly.

As she anticipated the final interview, she was conflicted about whether or not to disclose her illness. Her last boss knew about the diabetes—Melanie was already employed at the time of her diagnosis—and he was very supportive when it was necessary for her to take time off or delegate job responsibility.

Melanie has always exceeded her performance goals, but she's well aware that her disease impacts how she works. At times, she can't perform the way others might because of the fluctuations of her illness. Although she wanted to disclose her diabetes to get a feel for how her prospective boss might respond, she worried that disclosure might work against her.

Talking About It

If you decide to talk about your AD during a job interview, these guidelines can assist you:

Details to Reveal:

- Keep It Short and Simple (KISS). Know your facts, deliver a clear message—don't use complex medical jargon—and remain calm. This will minimize overreactions and maximize everyone's comfort level.

- Some women choose not to name their particular disease, because of common misconceptions about many ADs. Instead, they refer to it as a "chronic condition."

- Alternatively, naming the disease can make it more concrete and allow others to draw on their own experiences, creating a more shared understanding of what it means for you.

- Focus on your talents and strengths, not on what you can't do.

- Provide concrete examples of how your illness affects you at work, such as frequent doctors' appointments, trouble using your hands, or reduced ability to walk.

- Reassure your boss and co-workers that you are prepared to take care of your health, and that your illness will not inconvenience them.

Attitude to Project:

- Set the tone with your words and behavior. Keep the conversation unemotional and matter-of-fact.
- Remember that you control this message. Be as public as you must be, and as private as you want to be.
- Model your message in the way in which you want others to receive it. If you are positive and upbeat, that's what they'll take away with them.
- Make it clear that you are neither embarrassed nor ashamed about living with an AD—even if it isn't the truth.

Time to Disclose:

- Bring up your AD when it is clear that the prospective employer wants to hire you and you are in the job-negotiation phase. Treat it like any other personal factor.
- Discuss it in person, rather than by e-mail or phone, so that you have the opportunity to create an effective dialogue and to project a positive tone.

On the day of the final interview, Melanie opted to disclose. When she was offered the job, she responded by revealing her diabetes and explaining that it is mostly under control. She explained that she monitors herself regularly and is skilled in planning ahead in the unlikely event that she becomes too sick to work. She told her prospective boss that she might not to be able to attend some functions and might have to leave work early on occasion. She finished by saying that her organizational skills allow her to assure everyone concerned that she'll always meet her deadlines without burdening others.

The upshot? Melanie's new boss didn't have a problem with any of it, and he now gives her all the support she needs to take care of her health and perform her job successfully.

Many women believe it's in their best interest to disclose their AD before taking a job. Maybe they'll need special accommodations at some point down the road, so they choose to take a proactive stance and reveal their condition prior to hire. Some think that early disclosure reveals important information about the organization's attitude toward illness. Others simply feel better when they're up-front from the outset.

Choosing Not to Disclose During a Job Interview

Claudia, a graphic designer, lives with scleroderma. Because of weakness in her hands, she has trouble moving a mouse and using a keyboard. She has become very adept at using voice-recognition software (VRS), and can work almost as efficiently as she could with her hands. Claudia developed the disabling symptoms at her last job, where her boss and co-workers were very supportive. She believes it was easy for them to treat her as they always had because she had already proven her talents and her value to the agency.

Therefore, when Claudia took a job with a different design firm, she chose not to disclose the scleroderma until she had started working, although she made sure that the agency's equipment was compatible with her software. The first day, she installed her VRS and got straight to work. A few weeks later, in a meeting with her boss and her team, she told them that she had a health condition that periodically made it too difficult to use a mouse and she chose to use VRS all the time to keep her skills up.

One year later, when her boss was asked about how he reacted when he learned that Claudia worked this way, he acknowledged that he might not have hired her if he had known about the issues with her hands. However, he added that, within a few days of Claudia's arrival on the job, she had become an integral part of the team and no one had second thoughts about her hire.

In this case, Claudia's decision not to disclose during the hiring process worked in her favor. Even though she knew that she could do the job using VRS, she guessed that her boss might have had second thoughts—and her hunch was right. Claudia relied on her personal experience and her belief in her capabilities to make her decision about disclosure.

Her strategy was to seamlessly integrate the accommodations she needed to do the job and wait until she had proven her value before discussing her health issues. This also gave her time to gauge how others might respond to an employee's chronic health problems. And, when she disclosed, she didn't tell people individually because she felt that she would be more comfortable disclosing to everyone at once, keeping it on a professional level. Claudia knew her own comfort level and also understood what she believed were her best moves. This gave her the confidence she needed to show others that her health was not going to be a burden to anyone.

Unfortunately, there are situations in which disclosure will lead to more trouble than it's worth. But keep in mind that the problems that arise after disclosure might be averted with more careful attention to your own behavior. It's worth taking a good look at your situation and considering what is best for you, rather than blindly following the advice of others. When the symptoms of your condition impact your ability to perform the activities that your job requires, you're better off disclosing the situation.

Choosing to Disclose When You're Already Employed

The following suggestions give you a few ways to consider the issue of disclosure and some guidelines you can use toward developing your competence in talking about this very important subject.

What to Say

First, your biggest challenge is to describe something that other people have trouble understanding, particularly when your symptoms are vague. Statements like, "I'm sleepy because I'm in a flare" or "The MS is acting up again, and I'm dizzy" accurately represent fatigue, but they also describe conditions that people who don't have an AD also might feel. That's why it's important to focus your message on how the particular symptom affects *you*. Everyone feels sleepy at one time or another during a workday, but when *you're* sleepy, it goes a step beyond. You might find it difficult to focus on reading. You might need to sit rather than stand. You might even need to sneak off for a nap. Somehow, you need to make this distinction.

Then there's the fact that many AD symptoms are not apparent to others. Even those that we consider visible (such as facial stretching in scleroderma) can go completely unnoticed, even by those close to us. How do you express the numbness or stiffness in your hand that prevents you from holding a pencil? How do you explain the pain in your joints or muscles? How do you communicate a feeling to another person and be clearly understood?

You can start by describing the symptom and clarifying how it affects you *at the moment*. You might say: "My fingers feel numb and weak, and they aren't gripping properly because of (illness), so I can't hold a pen. I'll use my laptop to take notes until the condition improves." Or: "I

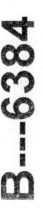

have sharp, shooting pain in my stomach because of (illness), and it gets worse when I walk. So, I'll avoid walking whenever possible today and ask people to meet in my office instead."

Finally, symptoms change—getting better or worse with little, if any, warning. If *you* find it confusing, imagine what it's like for co-workers who have no idea that a shift has taken place unless you tell them. That's a big "unless," because many of us find that explaining coming and going symptoms is the hardest part of communicating about our illnesses.

It's likely that you feel angry or disappointed when a symptom reappears or worsens. You want to scream at the world, or crawl into bed and hide. At times like these, it's very difficult to collect yourself and speak coherently about your situation to someone who is relying on you at work. Just remember to focus on the outcome of this change.

If a new symptom means that a task will be delayed, explain that there are times when you can't do certain things that you could do the day before. You might say something like: "I have to leave work this morning because I can't see well out of my left eye. I know I look the same as yesterday, but my productivity is compromised today."

Consider How Your Own Feelings Influence Your Message

We all have complicated feelings about living with illness, and this can affect what we say and how we say it. It also influences how we respond to the comments of others.

I've lived with multiple sclerosis (MS) for almost 30 years, and I'm still unsettled when I say to someone for the first time, "I have MS." While I'm not necessarily uncomfortable revealing this fact, I'm often thrown into self-consciousness by the reactions I get. You may be familiar with the excessive cluckings of sympathy…the thoughtless comments that reveal a lack of knowledge about the disease…the blank look, followed by a quick change of subject.

I've learned that I can't possibly prepare for the settings in which I find I'm disclosing this highly personal information. But I've also learned that I manage these situations better by understanding my own feelings and clearly articulating my own experience. This is when our warrior skills come into play, triggering our ability to stay focused and balanced and allowing us to communicate as we intend.

Consider How You Respond to Others

Let's start with the comments that reflect misunderstanding or ignorance. Many people are uneducated about autoimmune illness, even a common one such as MS. I've been asked if I was one of "Jerry's kids" (that's muscular dystrophy). A client with rheumatoid arthritis says she can't remember how often she's been asked, skeptically, how she can have such an affliction when she's not old (they're confusing it with osteoarthritis). Another, who has diabetes, finds that some people at work watch her like a hawk when she eats, making her feel as if she's in a fish bowl. Then there are those who are skeptical about illness that isn't acute (*"Aren't you better yet?"*) or where symptoms aren't obvious (*"How can you be sick when you look fine?"*). And let's not forget the well-meaning folks who have the perfect cure: *"Aunt Sue was cured by drinking kelp smoothies"* or *"My brother-in-law got better with massage."*

Fortunately...blessedly...others can communicate with sensitivity. If you live with AD, you know exactly what I mean. You also know that deciding whether or not to disclose an illness in the work world is an even more highly charged issue. Let's face it—how people respond can make the difference between whether or not you can do your job successfully.

Katherine is a retail store manager for a national home-goods chain. She started as a cashier 15 years ago, and steadily worked her way up the career ladder. Three years ago, she was diagnosed with mixed connective tissue disease (MCTD).

In the beginning, Katherine physically felt the same as she always had, and, for the most part, forgot about the diagnosis. She was taught that certain things, such as illness, are private and meant to be discussed very selectively. Besides, she didn't know what to say, since her own understanding of the disease was minimal. She decided that she would reveal it at work on a need-to-know basis. Since the symptoms were not affecting her, she disclosed only to a friend in human resources, with whom she discussed her corporate benefits.

If, while you are employed, you develop AD or your symptoms become worse, you can follow the same disclosure guidelines you would use when starting a new job. Just don't wait until the illness adversely affects your performance and puts your job in jeopardy.

If you don't need special accommodations, and your performance is unaffected, the timing for disclosure is your choice. You might decide to do it immediately, or wait until the symptoms become a problem. Ask yourself:

- Am I ready to talk about this with other people? (If you're feeling scared, overwhelmed, or angry, you might want to get used to the feelings before discussing your illness with others.)

- Have I had sufficient time to live with my AD, to learn how it will affect my body?
- Am I being realistic about what I hope to get from others?
- Do I know enough about this disease to discuss it competently?

Over the past year, Katherine developed heart problems as a result of the MCTD. She decided to learn more about the condition and, armed with this new information, changed some personal and work habits to try to stay healthy. Because she's more tired than she used to be and doesn't eat or drink the way she once did, she no longer socializes with co-workers. She rarely attends company dinner events, and quit both the bowling and softball leagues. She delegates more work than she used to, and she gives her assistant managers a lot more of the physical work than she used to.

Recently, a good friend revealed that the rumor mill claims that Katherine doesn't seem to be committed to the company any longer. The gossip is that she and her husband must be planning to start a family, or that she's looking for another job. What's more, her district manager has commented several times on her late reports.

Tips to Disclosing at Work When You Are Already Employed

- Determine who should be told. At first, it might be best to keep the information on a need-to-know basis, so that you don't run the risk of it becoming water-cooler gossip.
- Explain what has changed and why you are disclosing the AD now.
- Make it clear that you've waited to talk about it because:
  - You need an accommodation that requires a financial investment or a reorganization of systems and/or staff.
  - You want to do something differently so that the symptoms don't get in your way.
  - You're not asking for an accommodation, but you want to give your co-workers the courtesy of knowing that things have changed for you (for example, you're not as quick as you were, or you'll be taking some time off).
- Keep your explanation as simple as possible, particularly in the beginning, to allow yourself time to get more comfortable with talking about it at work. Know the facts—and stick to them.

- Remember that many people will need time to digest the news that you have a chronic illness. You might suggest that you're available to discuss their questions and concerns at a later time.

In one meeting, he told her that some of her co-workers were grumbling because she seems distracted and less willing to work as hard. And then he shared that he had been considering promoting her, but he's no longer sure that she's ready. Katherine felt increasingly isolated and confused, and didn't know what to do or to whom to turn. She considered finding a job with a lot less responsibility or applying for disability.

Unfortunately, this kind of situation is too common—and entirely unnecessary. Instead of trying to convince yourself, and everyone else, that your illness is not affecting your work, it's easier just to tell others what's going on. When disabling symptoms prevent you from delivering your best performance, you can ignore this fact for only so long. If you're struggling to get the job done because of medical appointments or time off due to illness, people will notice. If your mood is different, people will notice. Even if you're meeting your goals, people will wonder if something is wrong when your behavior and work style change. Unless you give them reason to think otherwise, they'll assume that you've become less motivated or unable to do the job—and you are likely to lose their support.

On the other hand, when you offer a reason that others can comprehend, you demonstrate that your commitment has not diminished—even in the face of changing abilities. Particularly when you've established a good reputation and created valuable relationships, most people will be willing to give you the support you need. Yes, your illness might not be "okay" with everyone, but disclosing it will go a long way toward maintaining your credibility.

Another factor to examine when considering disclosure is the risk of isolation. If you're feeling disconnected from your co-workers because they have no idea what you're going through, there's a good chance it's showing. Chronic illness is a significant part of your experience, and hiding it makes it much more difficult to stay fully integrated in the world. If your symptoms leave you with less energy or feeling depressed, discussing your situation can help you reconnect with others. But be careful not to complain about your situation, or make it the only thing you talk about.

As in Katherine's case, suffering or getting by in silence often leads to the loss of well-earned respect. Underperformance is attributed to lack of motivation, insufficient skills, or lack of interest, when it is really an admirable attempt at managing a difficult situation.

The bottom line is that it's too easy to lose valuable relationships and strong supporters because they don't know what you're going through, what you need, or how they can help. It's up to you to evaluate what's most important for your sense of self and ability to function well, and then to adapt your already honed relationship-building skills to create and maintain the support you need.

Ongoing Communication With People Who Already Know

Once you decide to be up-front about your condition, the communication isn't complete. Revealing an illness to your bosses or co-workers does not ensure that they will understand—or remember—how this impacts your work.

Communication Guidelines

By observing what people say or do that makes you uncomfortable, then developing responses that allow you to handle the situation with grace, you can learn how to effectively respond to the comments of others. Here are some guidelines:

Don't:

- Leave it up to others to form their own ideas about why you are doing your work differently.

- Assume people already know what they need to know about your situation and that, if they wanted to help, they would.

- Wait until you have underperformed so badly that no one believes you can succeed.

- Complain about your illness. Save that for confidential chats with your dog.

Do:

- Maintain a matter-of-fact attitude about your illness and its impact on you. Avoid drama, and interject humor whenever possible.

- Have a contingency plan to ensure that work gets done in a timely fashion in the event that you're having problems. Let others know, so they are clear about what they can expect.

- Be patient when others forget that you can't do something or question why your abilities today are different from yesterday. Becoming visibly upset only alienates others and compounds your problem.
- Stay focused on why you were hired in the first place: to get the job done and done well. You can do it, girlfriend.

On the days when you feel your worst, you can look fine. You don't sport the red nose of a cold or the cast of a broken wrist to support your case. Because you look the same as you do on your good days, you wonder if people understand the symptoms that they cannot see. Making things even more difficult, most of the physical challenges associated with an AD—such as fatigue, stomach problems, and pain—are regularly experienced by "healthy" folks. So, how do you explain that what you feel has a different dimension without sounding like a drama queen?

You might find that co-workers make incorrect assumptions about you because of your illness, thinking you are less capable than you actually are. Over time, this can lead to becoming marginalized or even underemployed. There are also those who make undesirable and unsolicited comments about your health. They ask how you're feeling when you're not in the mood to talk about it, or they comment that you're not looking so hot when you're feeling just fine. Others try to "help" with advice or stories about someone they know with the same illness that you have. Oh, for a pair of earplugs!

Furthermore, a chronic illness can become wearisome to others—it certainly is to you. In the beginning, people tend to respond with sympathy and support. But, as time goes by, they wonder why you aren't "better" by now. Most people have a short amount of patience for issues that don't get resolved. Sometimes, the most difficult responses are from those who have faced trauma themselves: *I got over it, why can't you?*

Then there is the "blame-the-victim" mentality. You must be making yourself sick because you're too anxious, stressed, or tightly wound. Ironically, I've heard stories in which the most difficult person to contend with is the person who also has a chronic illness. This can be very hard to comprehend, but, in fact, I liken it to the I-got-out-of-the-ghetto-why-can't-you mentality. Some people have a difficult time empathizing with others who don't seem to do as well as they do with what appears to be the same challenge.

In fact, you can manage this if you follow one simple guideline: don't refer to how you feel any more than is necessary. Your best bet is to speak about your symptoms only when you need an accommodation or have to explain something. Even the most empathetic person gets tired of hearing that you're not feeling well. You want to show others that you are managing the situation, and it is not—and will not be—their problem.

Competencies to Develop

Unfortunately, the world will always include people who respond to just about every new situation with negativity. And it's also home to perfectly reasonable folks who simply haven't a clue about what to say to you. But you can address these difficulties by looking for occasions to demonstrate that you are just as capable of getting the work done as anyone else, even if you handle it differently.

Communication is a challenge for a lot of people. That's why so many organizations make it a mandatory management course. Once again, we can see that living with AD means that we have to get good at the same stuff that everyone else struggles with. The context and the nuance might change, but the heart of each issue remains the same.

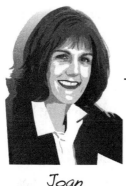

Joan

7

You're Fired—
By Your Body or
Your Boss

In June of 1992, at the age of 36, I was happily employed, married, and the mother of a 7-year-old child. I was very much at home in my dual role as store manager and regional training manager for a national bookstore chain. It was a dream job, and I was steadily moving up the company ladder.

Suddenly, acute bowel symptoms took me down. Continuous bleeding, anemia, intense cramping, and weight loss landed me in the hospital a few weeks later. Little did I know, it would be the beginning of a long journey of discovery and adjustment.

While in the hospital, I was promoted to acting district manager (neither my employer nor I anticipated that this would be a long-term illness). Several months—and one more disability and hospitalization—later, a new district manager was hired. Shortly after a company merger, I lost my training position and someone new took over my region, largely because the condition of my store suffered as a result of the additional responsibility I took on while dealing with my illness. Needless to say, I was crushed. I loved training and had a very hard time dealing with the loss of my position.

A few months later, I left the company in search of new opportunities. I landed a store-manager position with another retail company—and hated it. Finding an office position was next on my list, since I hoped my years of retail management would translate effectively into the corporate environment. I was eventually offered a job, but it wasn't in management. Instead, my new role was that of executive assistant to a successful business owner and leader.

Within a year, I had another flare-up and was out on disability for 10 days. The day after my return to the office, I was let go because "things weren't working out." In other words: I was fired! I'd never been fired before, and my reaction was one of bewilderment and dismay.

I might have gone to court to fight the termination, but I decided not to. Instead, I leveraged the relationships I'd developed with other leaders in the business community to find my next job (by then I was divorced and a single mom, so finding a new job was imperative). I was lucky enough to have a lot of support among local professionals, so it took only a couple of weeks to land another position—ironically, with the help of the company that had let me go. It was also the beginning of a 4-year odyssey, punctuated by times of wellness and times of illness. Throughout all the ups and downs, I continued to examine my priorities as I made my way through three more jobs.

Each disability leave became an opportunity to re-evaluate my direction. Whenever I became ill, I took it as a sign that I needed to make more adjustments. It seemed imperative to figure out what my heart and my body needed to be productive and healthy. I can now look back upon the demotion and firing with some objectivity, but, at the time, they shook my confidence and caused me to question my abilities.

Although posing a temporary setback—if you call 4 years temporary—these events also served as catalysts in the search for my true career calling. After I was fired, I took a long, hard look at what I really wanted to do with my professional life. I read a book called *Do What You Are* by Paul D. Tieger and Barbara Barron-Tieger, which makes career recommendations based on the Myers-Briggs personality assessment (1). Career counseling was one of the options suited to my personality type, and I found myself attracted to it. Despite everything, I was very good at getting jobs—and I certainly knew what it was like to navigate transitions.

Five jobs, one firing, one divorce, a new marriage, and six rounds of disability leave later, I was ready to leave the corporate world to start my coaching business. It took almost 7 years to get to that point, and another 2 to take the leap.

To this day, I believe that my decision to start a coaching business was one of the best things I could have done for myself. It is certainly among the top five factors that have positively affected my ability to continue working, make the most of my talents and experience, and tend to the needs of my body. It hasn't always been easy—and there are days when I've worked from bed—but it's been right for me. Perhaps it might also be right for you.

The Nudge

As with many life-altering events, an autoimmune illness is almost guaranteed to cause you to re-evaluate your priorities. Many women I've met have said that this is one of the gifts embedded in the challenge. Options and opportunities they might never have considered suddenly became possible—and desirable.

Terri is divorced with two children, one of whom has a fairly severe disability. She shares a home with her mother— a decision that allows her to put a roof over her children's heads and share parenting. She's a talented musician and songwriter, but her dream of becoming a star was muted by obligations, the endometriosis she battled, the environmental sensitivities that affect her, and the years she lost as a result.

When I met Terri, she had just begun to get out again after 18 months of staying close to home and spending a lot of time in bed. I didn't know it at the time, but her attendance at my workshop was one of the first things she did once she had the energy to leave the house for more than an hour at a time. She was terrified that the only way she could support her children was to go back to work full time, and she was sure she couldn't do so, given her need for frequent rest. She had no idea what other options might enable her to earn a living without compromising her health. She was still financially linked to her ex-husband, but she was finally well enough to consider breaking the ties.

Sometime during the workshop series, Terri got "the nudge." She realized that she does have a choice, and she might be able to generate income without going back to a boring, stressful job. She came up with the idea to utilize her talents as a musician to start a music-lesson business for young people in her neighborhood. She didn't know what that would take or exactly how she would do it, but she felt that she could be successful…that she could make enough money to sever her dependence on her ex-husband and have the ability to set her own hours so that she could take care of herself and her boys.

In most cases, the nudge causes you to start asking yourself a series of practical questions. You may not choose to act right away, remaining for a while longer in the trauma phase accompanied by bewilderment, pain, and fear. But when you emerge and move into acceptance and stabilization, you may consider self-employment an attractive choice—just as Terri did, and just as many others have done.

Self-Employment—Practical Matters For Everyone

Self-employment or business ownership is risky, even for a healthy person, so it might seem to be a downright ridiculous choice for a woman who's also dealing with the symptoms of a chronic illness. Truthfully, self-employment has an inherent set of opportunities and risk factors, no matter what your circumstances. Pros and cons must be considered by anyone who is contemplating such a career move, and then the fluctuations of autoimmune disease (AD) must be tossed into the equation. Let's look at the common factors first.

The Entrepreneurial Personality—Fact or Fiction?

Open any book about business ownership, and you're likely to see a checklist or questionnaire to help you determine if you have the qualities required to be a successful business owner. Consequently, the first step is to figure out if you possess those qualities.

To be sure, specific personality traits—innovative, aggressive/assertive, take-charge—are readily associated with the "innate" entrepreneur, but the absence of these qualities does not disqualify you from successful self-employment. For starters, your goals for self-employment—to remain a gainfully employed, engaged woman who needs to modify her lifestyle in order to take care of her body and family and/or enjoy a decent social life—may be different from the objectives of the individual for whom excitement and wealth may be motivating factors.

According to Paul and Sarah Edwards, who have written several books for home-based business owners, "The majority of people who start home-based businesses are not 'innate' entrepreneurs (2)." In fact, the

National Survey of Entrepreneurial Parents, a study co-sponsored by the authors, revealed that 74% of the 606 people surveyed came from corporate positions (3). Changing circumstances associated with children and family were a greater factor in their choices than the pure desire to create something on their own.

Candace is in business for herself, although she did not originally set out to be an entrepreneur. Instead, she stumbled into it upon returning to work after being severely sick from autoimmune hepatitis and finding herself out of a job. A successful mortgage broker, she discovered that she could easily work from home. Aside from the need to affiliate herself with a brokerage firm for the purpose of licensing, she was free to run her business as she saw fit. In addition to her many years in the industry, the foundation of her success was a strong work ethic and commitment to excellent service.

It has taken Candace a while to realize that she's in charge—free to make decisions about the hours she works, the kind of marketing strategies she employs, and the standards by which she runs her business. She has a strong need for financial security, which initially led her to take on too many loans at once and conflicted with her desire to spend more time with her growing family. She also had a hard time trusting people to perform to her standards, so she struggled with delegating responsibilities, even if it often meant performing additional tasks that she didn't especially like to do.

But Candace persisted. Along the way, she decimated at least 10 beliefs and rules she had previously embraced about "the way things are done in a successful business." One by one, she tackled them and tossed out those that were getting in her way.

It's been 4 years since I met Candace, and she's still going strong. She brought her husband into the business for a while, then decided that didn't work so well. Now she's partnered with someone who is really good at doing those things that Candace prefers to avoid. And, at a time when many mortgage firms are closing their doors, Candace has successfully opened up a new market in construction loans, which she finds exciting and fun.

Knowing that you don't have to be an innate entrepreneur is comforting, especially if self-employment is an attractive alternative to a nine-to-five job. Nonetheless, in the five plus years I've spent working with self-employed professionals—the majority of whom work from home—I've noticed several traits that make success possible.

Self-Starting

Even though you may possess a strong amount of initiative, you'll have little ability to demonstrate or exercise it when you're ill. And, if you happen to be a self-starter by nature, you'll probably feel extremely frustrated when your body demands that you slow down. Fortunately, this quality gives you the capacity to pick yourself up and get started again when you're able.

Being a self-starter is an essential component of self-employment, because the ups and downs, the necessary cycles of success and failure (I prefer to call them "learning experiences") require the ability to reboot even when you may not feel like it.

If you've been at a job for a long time, even one with a lot of independence, it's very different being out on your own. Suddenly, no one is there to tell you when to start your workday and when to end. It's completely up to you to decide how to spend your time, determine your priorities, and get the necessary work done.

One of the first things realized by those who leave the more structured company environment and choose this path is that they feel a little funny about their freedom.

Candace says she still remembers the exhilaration she felt the first week on her own—followed by the odd sensation of guilt, then fear. No boss dictated how her hours should be spent...when she could take off for lunch, when she could leave for home. All aspects of the business were firmly in her hands—and it felt strange. She was a self-starter all right, but she was used to deadlines imposed by someone else. She feared that, without the pressure imposed by a supervisor, she'd completely lose her motivation—and her business. In the past, the demands of others helped keep her in check. Now it was all up to Candace.

In truth, it was an absurd belief—considering that service and security were among her top five values—but it drove her nonetheless. Unfortunately, it caused her to work too much, which was not good for her health. To combat the growing problem, she hired a coach to help her work more effectively. Eventually, she learned how to work fewer hours with the confidence that she wasn't "falling down on the job."

Influencing

Defined as the ability to sway the will or behavior of others, being an influencer may sound sinister. However, it takes on a negative quality only if it's used for purposes that are less than noble. Technically, influencing people is the ability to communicate and connect, and it often requires a strong sense of confidence. As such, it's a characteristic that can be acquired.

The first year Heather ventured out on her own as a small-business consultant, and before she quit her full-time job, she knew she had to go out and solicit business. Unfortunately, she was frozen in her tracks and didn't make a move for several months. She remembers writing up a telephone script so that she'd have some guidelines about what to say if anyone called. Despite her desire to get her business off the ground, she was terrified that people would call—so afraid, in fact, that she often willed her phone not to ring. Despite having the skills to be a successful consultant, she lacked the knowledge and confidence in her ability to talk to people about what she does for a living.

Eventually, Heather figured out that she needed to learn the "language of influence"—otherwise known as marketing. Over the next few years, she took several courses that taught her how to share information about her profession. Her insecurities gradually diminished, and now she can engage in business conversations with complete ease. Taking this accomplishment a step further, she currently teaches classes in marketing so that she can help others gain the knowledge and skills to talk to people about their services with confidence and effectiveness.

The ability to influence others is valuable in other ways, as well. In the light of your illness, it's important to be able to talk to your family, gain their support, and ask for their help at times. If you hire someone to help you—such as a bookkeeper, business assistant, or housekeeper—you must be able to influence them to get things done to your standards. Exerting influence is a necessary quality of leadership when you are self-employed. We all have the ability to do it—some are just better at it than others. If you feel that it's not one of your strong suits, many programs and classes can help you gain the skill you need.

Organized and Focused

When you add organization and focus to the requisite bag of traits, you have a powerful combination. These can sometimes be elusive components, thrown off track by factors such as:

- More ideas than the time to implement them
- A feeling that the work is never really done
- Difficulty understanding priorities
- The pull of external distractions and demands (family, house chores, e-mail)
- Responsibility for multiple business functions (customer service, order fulfillment, marketing,

administration, invoicing and record keeping, deliverables)

The trick is to develop systems and structures, and to involve team members who can help you with organization and focus. Business ownership requires you to wear more hats than most people need at a job so, even if you possess these skills, having others around to ease your burden can make a big difference. Paying attention to the details and keeping priorities in check is critical to staying afloat.

When Danielle first started out on her own as a photographer, she had very few time boundaries and little control over her schedule. She worked 7 days a week, and her hours frequently spilled into the evening and beyond. Because she didn't think she could afford employees and feared handing over any work, she did everything on her own.

Tired of having no time to enjoy the rest of her life, Danielle hired a coach. After taking that first step, she hired a full-time assistant, a part-time assistant, and an accountant. Now she's much more comfortable with delegating and, even though she still has work to do in this area, her skills have greatly improved. She now takes every Sunday as a personal day—without exception. She has all the business she needs, and can begin to devote time to the creative work she loves because she can count on the team she has assembled.

Dedicated and Persistent

Building a successful business is a process. While it's definitely exciting and fulfilling, it's also accompanied by a host of challenges and learning experiences. Your limits will be tested, and you'll frequently be called upon to push even harder and march on as you face the challenges that accompany business ownership. Without dedication and persistence, you'd probably give up when any one of the possible obstacles came up to bite you in the face.

Lorraine has lived with fibromyalgia for nearly 15 years. For 10 of those years, she has tried to forge a successful business that would allow her to support herself and manage the ups and downs of her illness.

She had previously worked in marketing for a few small, start-up, high-tech firms, but she could no longer maintain the pace. As an alternative, Lorraine started selling a friend's handmade jewelry out of her home. In time, she found other jewelry makers who wanted her to market their pieces, and it wasn't long before she'd built a tidy little business.

Unfortunately, Lorraine wasn't making quite enough to live comfortably and afford health insurance. When the Internet started to take off, she used her technology background and contacts to learn the skills she needed to set up a Web site and sell jewelry on eBay.® After several months and a small investment, she found that this option was even less lucrative because of the small markup. What's more, it was physically exhausting to photograph all the pieces and ship them to customers.

Lorraine soon discovered that a need existed for people who could train others on how to profit by using the Internet. Over the past 3 years, her business has grown by 50% annually, and she sees many other opportunities on the horizon.

Flexible and Adaptive

If you are inflexible and have difficulty adapting to what comes your way (lacking failure-recovery skills), you may stubbornly refuse to alter course when all signs suggest that you should. Of course, if you're dealing with AD, you may already have been forced to develop these qualities, even if they're not in your nature. However, innate behavior is quirky. Even if one set of circumstances requires you to learn new behaviors, an innate quality may still influence you in other situations, requiring you to build your "flexibility muscles" all over again.

Above all else, flexibility and adaptability increase your chances of persisting in the face of setbacks and changing direction when you realize that something you're doing is not working. Remember Heather? After more than 5 years in her own business, she can attest to this fact.

Heather's fourth year was her worst ever, and she made only as much money as she did when employed as a retail clerk nearly 20 years ago. She realized that she had to refocus her attention and redouble her efforts to get her business back on track. It meant swallowing some pride, asking for help, and seeking contract work to rebuild her foundation quickly; she did what was necessary to move forward. The upshot? Heather's fifth year was the best to date, and year six is proving to shape up as another period of growth, as well.

Innovative

Innovation is a sister of flexibility and adaptability, and it can be the killer of organization and focus. How's that for a double-edged sword? Nonetheless, if, for example, you've been in the corporate world and are thinking about taking some key talents and skills from those experiences to start your own business, you're already demonstrating the quality of innovation. It's at play when you figure out what those skills are, and when you develop a way to convert them into a business of your own. It's at play when you figure out how to market a service or sell products in such a way that others can see the value—and they're happy to pay for it.

Elizabeth is the author of a popular marketing book, as well as a speaker and trainer. She identified her target market and niche at the start of her business and was an early adopter of many of the systems and tools now used by other service professionals who make money from their core expertise. She admits that she has more exciting ideas than she'll ever have time to implement, but fortunately, she's practical.

To stop herself from wasting time and energy on projects that would be more distracting than productive, she's learned to accept the fact that she simply can't do everything that's on her creative agenda. Over time, she has developed a set of criteria to help her evaluate her goals, the first of which is keeping profitable projects afloat. In addition, she has established a minimal-income standard for any project she undertakes. By employing these methodologies, her innovation has served her well, enabling her to build her business with a great deal of success.

The Pros and Cons of Being Self-employed

Any good act of due diligence would suggest creating a list of pros and cons, no matter what options you're weighing. Pros and cons exist with any choice, and it's critical to be aware of both sides of the equation to get a realistic picture and gain the ability to make an informed choice.

The chart on the next page lists the pros and cons of being a self-employed professional working from home. The data have been collected through direct experience and the observations of business experts. This information would be true for anyone considering self-employment, regardless of the circumstances.

As you review the lists, you may be intrigued by some items and disturbed by others. Fair enough. To determine if this new undertaking is right for you, I recommend a SWOT analysis: strengths, weaknesses, opportunities, and threats. Using SWOT as a model, it's likely that the exciting elements of self-employment tap into your strengths or represent opportunities. Those that cause your stomach to flip-flop probably point to weaknesses or sound off alarms of fear.

Pros and Cons of Being Self-Employed

Pros	Cons
You can work from home in a comfortable and controllable environment—pajamas optional.	Working from home means distractions, such as children, housecleaning, and—dare I say it?—"Oprah."
You're the boss.	As the boss, you need a great deal of focus and tenacity to get important things done.
There's no commute.	You might work more hours than you normally would, since your job is always right under your nose.
No one dictates your stop and start times.	Without others to report to, your sense of discipline may be reduced.
The expenses associated with commuting, eating out, and business attire are reduced or eliminated.	You are solely responsible for all business and equipment expenses.
The pressure of company and management deadlines is nonexistent.	If you enjoy the stimulation of others around you, you might get lonely.
You might be able to work fewer hours and make the same amount of money.	You'll leave the comfort zone of a steady paycheck.

You can make money doing something you enjoy and do well.	You'll have to take charge of sales and marketing, which are critical to your success.
You're available to your children and for other appointments—within limits.	You might have to endure the background noise of family life and a lack of privacy when you need to focus.
You can include family members in your business.	You might have to rely on the help of family members when, in fact, paid staff would be more reliable.
You can get significant tax advantages.	You could possibly experience issues with health insurance in the face of your pre-existing condition.

If you think self-employment or business ownership would be a good alternative, you can use SWOT to figure out how to make the most out of the factors that are advantageous to you, and how to deal with those that are difficult. Rather than hoping and praying—or hiding your head in the sand—you can develop strategies to address your weaknesses and potential threats up front.

When I started managing my business full-time, I was one happy camper. Finally, I could set my own hours and establish my own pace. I could work in natural light without air conditioning—which seemed to aggravate my symptoms—from the comfort of home. If I needed more time in the morning—in the bathroom—I could take it without fear of embarrassment. I could interact with clients when the time was right for me, and I could make more money per hour than I did "on the job." Perhaps best of all, I could utilize a wide range of skills that I enjoyed, giving me an emotional boost that I didn't always experience when working for someone else.

When I first left the corporate world, I was feeling pretty good physically. My symptoms were minimal and manageable. I had the support of my husband and income from a handful of paying clients. I was ready to take on more, and I had mastered the basic marketing conversations.

If I were to review the pros and cons list today, I'd embrace all but one of the pros—I don't hire family members. Some of the cons would have threatened me, so I'd have to deal with the impact of about two or three of them.

That's where the SWOT analysis comes in handy. Once you've identified your weaknesses and potential threats, you can more readily address them. If you can do so effectively, and the pros outweigh the cons, you stand a good chance of success.

Self-Employment and Business Ownership With Autoimmune Disease

It doesn't matter how creative or skilled you are—when you're dealing with acute symptoms of your illness, the majority of your energy is needed for basic survival and healing. As such, it's not a good time to start a business. However, when your body has thrown you in bed, remanded you to the sofa, or landed you in the hospital, you may begin to think about self-employment. It just might be a lucrative way to earn your keep, contribute something to the world, and have more control over your schedule.

As mentioned earlier, never before has there been greater flexibility in the workplace, and the same is true for owning and running a business. The Internet, reduced phone costs, and constantly evolving technology have opened up countless doors of opportunity for those who are considering self-employment. In fact, these days, it's even possible to

◇◇◇◇◇◇◇◇◇◇◇◇◇◇◇◇◇◇◇◇◇◇◇◇◇◇◇◇◇◇◇◇◇◇

Businesses You Can Conduct by Phone

Keep in mind that all of these businesses would require some computer time, since e-mail, database systems, and basic business structures are best managed with technology.

- Training (tele-classes)
- Consulting
- Coaching
- Network marketing

Businesses You Can Run From Your Computer:

- eBay® online store
- Amazon.com® online store
- Desktop publishing
- Web design
- Online sales of information products
- Writing and publishing

Businesses You Can Run from Your Kitchen and/or Kitchen Table:

- Catering
- Baking
- Gift baskets
- Direct sales

Businesses You Can Run from Bed:

- Anything you can do by phone
- Anything you can do on the computer

launch an online business using other people's products to make your fortune.

Turning Limitations into Strategies

Make a list of your strengths, weaknesses, opportunities, and threats as you see them today. Of course, they will change over time, but tackling this step is a fundamental part of your due diligence. By taking a good look at your present limitations—and any that may arise over time—you can begin to think about ways in which to address them. Essentially, this is a SWOT analysis for your health, and it allows you to develop strategies for overcoming issues that might hamper your success.

Several years ago, I met Stacy, a successful business consultant whose symptoms of type I diabetes posed only a periodic problem. I made her acquaintance a few months before the onset of my first signs of AD, so I didn't fully understand the challenges she faced. Some days, relaxing quietly was her best option. On other days, I'd call to discover that she was pedaling away on her stationary bike. Because of her illness, her energy and strength would ebb and flow unpredictably.

Rather than surrender to her illness, she came up with creative ways to handle her fluctuating symptoms, increase her stamina, and continue to be productive. She worked from

A Few Ways to Get You Moving in the Right Direction

- Consider your hobbies. What kinds of things do you do in your free time that you really enjoy?
- Review your résumé. Look for common themes and specialized knowledge.
- Talk to your best friends, trusted colleagues, and family members. Ask them to define your top five skills, and look for common responses.
- Think about the roles you play with your family and friends. Are you the organizer, the confidante, the bookkeeper? Odds are, you'll identify a pattern here, too.

Ask Yourself:

- What kinds of things are easy for you to do, but that others find difficult?
- What do you dream about doing, but haven't dared to try—until now?
- What activities are you engaged in when time just flies by?
- What would you do even if no one paid you to do it?

home, and her bed often served as an office when she needed to be particularly comfortable. She used a telephone headset to reduce physical stress, long before it was widely available.

Depending on your illness, you'll have different limitations to consider, both now and in the future. If your illness impacts your nervous system and affects the use of your hands and arms, a computer-based business may not be your best solution. The same would be true if your eyesight or attention span were compromised. Instead, a business that involves more phone time might be a smarter choice.

If you're toying with the idea of a business—such as corporate consulting or training—that requires you to get up and out early and commute to a customer's work site, and your illness requires you to stay close to the bathroom, you might want to rethink things. However, if your strengths are such that this is a lucrative solution, you might opt to partner with others who can fill in and give you flexibility on bad days. Alternatively, you could focus on material development while a partner delivers the training.

You've Finally Decided—Now What?

When you make the decision to set out on your own, there are many factors to address. If you've felt the nudge, you may already have some idea of what you might do. The following steps are not meant to be comprehensive, but rather to highlight some of the basics of going solo. As your business grows and different issues arise, you can revisit them and make new decisions or directional shifts.

Evaluate Your Skill Set

The quickest and easiest way to launch a business is to build on something you're already good at. When you choose a business that utilizes your talents and skills and suits your personality, you accomplish two things: you start off with a basic level of confidence in yourself, and you significantly reduce the time it takes to launch your business and make money. When your health is compromised, the fewer obstacles between you and your goal, the better!

So, what's the first step? Take a look at the skills you've developed on the job and in volunteer activities. Many of them can be just as valuable in your own business. Think about hobbies or dormant interests that just might have money-making potential. Scores of books and magazines are teeming with inspiring stories of women who have done just that.

Start by identifying your top five skills—a task that comes easier to some than to others. If you're humble

Earning Money

- Is there a need for your products or services? If so, who would be most likely to want what you're offering? Is there enough need and interest for you to make a living?
- What tools, systems, and resources will you need to perform your work, fulfill orders, respond to inquiries, organize your files, and follow up with people you meet?
- How will you deliver your services or products?
- How much will you charge people, and precisely what will they receive in return?
- How will you let others know what business you're in so that they can decide if they want what you offer or if they know people to whom they can refer you?
- What kind of marketing materials will you need to give people information about what you do and encourage them to buy?

by nature and aren't feeling particularly well, you may be hard-pressed to identify your unique talents and embrace them as valuable. But that doesn't mean you don't have any! It simply means you might need a bit of help in acknowledging them. Review the sidebar for some ideas to get you moving in the right direction.

Write down all the ideas you come up with. And, whatever you do, don't start worrying about making money—yet. I can't tell you how many times I've heard about a woman's explorations and musings grinding to a screeching halt because of premature money worries. For now, just remember that there are no bad ideas when brainstorming.

If you can't seem to shake your militant censor, get jump-started by purchasing a copy of the book *Brag! The Art of Tooting Your Own Horn without Blowing It* by Peggy Klaus (4). The author poses 12 questions that guide you through an exploration of your life, so that you can start to acknowledge—and love—your talents.

Do Some Market Research

Once you've identified your top five skills, it's time to package them to start your business. Is that panic I sense rising up in your belly? Fear not. There are probably more ways to build a business around your talents than you'll ever be able to accomplish. All you have to do is figure out which one would be most interesting and feasible, given what you know, need, and want. Look at the adjacent list to get some ideas about how to start earning money.

Next, you'll need a business plan, which can be either detailed or simple. Some folks won't make a move without one, while others will start first and get to the plan later. Either way, to get some real traction, a basic business plan can go a long way toward helping you understand your priorities, forecast your revenue and expenses, and identify your mission to help shape your marketing.

For a practical, easy-to-follow, and comprehensive book on the topic, pick up a copy of another of the Edwards' books, *Getting Business to Come to You* (5). For a fun and effective read, take a look at *The One Page Business Plan* (6). Set up like a children's workbook, it makes this daunting task much easier to tackle.

Sometimes, self-employed professionals would rather do anything than market their business, only to discover that, without an effective strategy, there *is* no business. While the need to tout your product or service may be obvious, it's the *level* of marketing that often surprises people—especially those who build their initial customer base through word of mouth. This luck factor can be very encouraging at the beginning, but, in time, a more proactive stance is required.

The biggest mistake most people make when it comes to marketing is deciding that it takes a certain personality to be successful. That is simply not true. Sure, you have to be able to communicate and come across as a decent human being, but beyond that, your success is more dependent on understanding the impact of various strategies, learning to speak the language of marketing, and determining the kinds of exposure that are most effective. For an easy-to-follow, yet extremely effective tool to help with marketing if you decide to start a service business, take a look at *Get Clients Now!* by C.J. Hayden (7).

If your energy is low, and you need plenty of time for rest, you can still be productive and successful—but you'll have to be smart about how you do your marketing. This brings me to the second biggest mistake people make when they think about marketing a business, and that's the erroneous belief that only a few ways exist for you to accomplish this task. Wrong.

In truth, there are probably 100 different ways to market a business. Your job is to figure out which of those marketing activities you would most enjoy doing (enjoyment goes a long way toward making you effective), and to understand their impact on your target clients. If you have only 1 hour a day to devote to marketing, or even just 3 hours a week, you can do it. Given such limited time, however, it stands to reason that you should concentrate your efforts on strategies that you enjoy and can handle—and that are also effective.

Once Terri made the decision to teach piano to young people from her home, she focused on two things: how to get the word out, and how to structure her time. She still needed plenty of rest, and she was not all that excited about marketing, but she knew it was important. Fortunately, she lives in a fairly affluent, family-oriented neighborhood—a fact that strongly influenced her decision to start the business. By running ads in the homeowners' newsletter and strategically placing fliers within the community, it was relatively easy to let her neighbors know what she was doing. Before long, Terri was receiving calls from interested parents.

As a songwriter and musician, her credibility was already high, and offering lessons locally was a plus. Given the nature of her business and the fact that her target market was nearby, her simple strategies were very effective. It took Terri just a couple of months to get her business well underway.

If Necessary, Compile a Team

Once you've noted your skills and identified the nature and focus of your business—and any physical limitations you need to tackle—it's time to think about how to address any gaps you might uncover. There's nothing more stressful than taking on more than you can handle, and you certainly don't need more of that.

When you have AD, it's easy to feel limited and holed up in a dark box if you're out of sorts for long periods of time. But when you face those limitations head on and think about what you need to do to move forward in spite of them, suddenly the walls of the box aren't as solid.

Many people aren't good at asking for help, and reasons vary from feeling less than deserving to not wanting to bother others. This hesitancy takes on an added dimension when you've been ill for a while, and you may believe that people are tired of being there for you (and the fact is that some of them may truly be worn a bit thin). But when you're launching a new business, the help you seek is of a completely different kind. This is not the time for your Lone Ranger persona to kick in—besides, even he had Tonto.

When you work for a company, you usually have a team of people performing various business functions. When you set out on your own, you are *all* those people. This isn't an impossible situation, and many people start out doing just about everything themselves. However, if you're not good at an essential business function or don't have the capacity to do everything, your best move is to bring in business partners to accomplish some of these jobs. You might benefit from hiring people (requiring an extra set of business activities such as payroll tax filings for compliance purposes) or from outsourcing certain functions to other professionals.

Self-employed professionals usually need to hire or contract with others to fulfill the following positions and responsibilities:

- CPA/accountant, bookkeeper, tax preparer
- Attorney/prepaid monthly legal package
- Scheduler
- Web designer and/or administrator
- Shopping-cart administrator
- Desktop publisher, copywriter
- Marketing assistant or professional
- Administrative assistant/virtual assistant (The latter, similar to an administrative assistant, runs a business from home and has multiple clients. Communication with a virtual assistant is done via e-mail, phone, and the Internet.)

With technology and the growing trend toward the use of 1099 subcontractors, finding the right people for your team is easier than ever before. Previously, self-employed professionals felt that they could hire help only if they were able to commit a certain number of hours a week for some of the more common positions, such as administrative assistant or book-keeper. These days, for a bit more per hour, you can hire specialists who are also in business for themselves. They don't need to invade your home, they are often more committed to excellence, and they are certainly more efficient because they're focused on specialized skill sets. Although their per-hour charges are usually higher than those of a full-time employee, you might be surprised to learn how much they can accomplish in just a few hours each month.

If you have teens in your family, or a spouse with some of the skills you need, you might want to draw them into your business. Although I've never done it, I know many who have. Treating them like any other employee—including reasonable pay, proper training, and clear expectations—can go a long way toward making this a viable solution.

Put the Right Systems in Place

I'd be remiss if I didn't mention the potential value of some commonly used systems that can be effective tools for simplification and automation. We usually think that delegation is done only through people, but that simply doesn't hold true in the twenty-first century. With the advent of auto-reply e-mail, online ordering and Internet shopping carts, e-newsletters, online calendars, and database-management tools, your ability to streamline many of your business processes can save you both time and money. Of course, if you're technologically challenged, you may need to get someone else to do the research and initial set-up. However you accomplish the task, these high-tech systems can definitely work to your advantage.

Explore the Issue of Health Insurance

Perhaps one of the major—and very legitimate—concerns about the self-employment alternative is access to sufficient, affordable health insurance. Some states require that all residents, regardless of health status, have access to health insurance. While that works in theory, it's an expensive proposition. And, despite the high cost, the coverage isn't always great. I know this first hand.

For a couple of years, my husband and I were both self-employed. After his COBRA ran out from his previous employer, we had to get medical insurance on our own. (COBRA, which stands for Consolidated Omnibus Budget Reconciliation Act, gives you

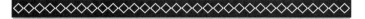

Healthcare Options and Other Issues

Depending on the business you choose, you're likely to find a professional organization that offers insurance—including group packages—for your particular field. The trick will be to find policies that operate in your favor regarding coverage and pre-existing conditions.

The Allied Service Worker's Union that provided my insurance serves self-employed professionals in Southern California. You can reach the company by mail at 22365 Barton Road, Suite 102, Grand Terrace, CA 92313, or by phone at 909.824.2180. It will take some research, but if you think that self-employment is an attractive option, by all means, look for other unions and organizations that offer health coverage to their members.

At the time of this writing, universal health insurance is not available to all citizens of the United States, and it is a topic of much debate. As one of millions of Americans with a chronic illness, you are deeply impacted by this. To find information and to look for ways that you, your family, and your friends can actively support initiatives in the legislature, search online using keywords such as "universal health insurance legislation."

coverage, at group rates, under your employer's insurance for 18 months after you lose your job or quit. In most cases, it will cost more than when you worked for the company, because you have to pay the entire premium, but it often costs less than individual insurance.) It was easy to find affordable insurance for my husband, but not for me. I could not even qualify for the coverage offered by the National Association for Self Employed (NASE) because of my pre-existing conditions and my relative state of health at the time.

Fortunately, I found coverage within a couple of months after the termination of COBRA benefits. The representative at NASE gave me contact information for the Allied Service Worker's Union. I received full coverage through an HMO, and the monthly rate wasn't too much of a stretch. It was certainly more affordable than paying the cash price for my doctor visits and the medicines required to manage my symptoms.

The downside was the annual increase in coverage costs, which came to about $100 more per month every year. But it's a price I'm willing to pay to be able to stay self-employed. I've always intended to make enough money in business to cover the cost of my insurance.

I certainly don't pretend to have the answer to the very important question of how to provide health-insurance coverage when you're working on your own. Like many things in life, it's a personal choice. However, I can pose a few questions to get you thinking about how to handle this issue:

- Can you come up with a business idea that leverages your talents and resources so that you can generate enough revenue to pay for sufficient health insurance?
- How would you weigh the possible health benefits of being self-employed with the financial security of having a job with good coverage? What other factors come into play here?
- If you stay at a job for the medical benefits, is it because you can't afford to get coverage on your own, or are you putting limits on your choices out of fear and lack of information?

The decision to make the transition from working for a company to self-employment is a personal one, and it can be precipitated by any number of factors. While I can't give you a magic formula for making this choice, I hope I've helped you understand some of the most common factors to consider in case you feel the nudge. More than anything, I want you to know that if you choose to keep working and think you might be happier, more fulfilled, and better served by self-employment, *you can do it.* Rosalind and I are right there with you, as are the many other women who have gone before you.

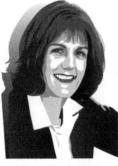

Joan

8

Building Your Support Team

It's undeniably true: your illness has changed the way you view your world and your life. It has quite literally transformed your physical capabilities—at least for the short term—and has most likely altered your perception of yourself. Depending on your orientation to the world before the onset of your symptoms, you may have discovered strengths you didn't know you had or frailties you wish you didn't have. Either way, this is not the time to go it alone.

When you are ill and navigating the numerous changes in your life, the process becomes infinitely easier if you have a strong circle of support. This chapter is intended to help you develop that circle... to help you put together the team that will give you maximum support and empowerment. We'll consider factors such as:

- Who can help you?
- What qualities are required of your team members?
- What attitude and level of compassion do you need to develop for yourself to make the best of this difficult situation?

You may be surprised to discover that the various members of your team will have a crossover effect on many aspects of your life. Co-workers may help you develop personal coping mechanisms. Family members may provide strategies to assist in the workplace. And the medical professionals who support you—doctors, complementary health specialists, and the like—can be great allies regarding work issues.

As you think about your team, keep in mind that illness—especially long-term chronic illness—is a tricky thing. It can distort your mental and emotional responses, making it difficult to figure out who to tell and what to disclose. As Rosalind has stated, even after 30 years, she remains conscious of the varying responses when she reveals her multiple sclerosis to someone new. You'll need to have the same mental preparedness, girlfriend—especially at times when you're feeling vulnerable and weak.

When you're in pain, it's not always easy to be discerning. You may not even know how you really feel about your illness or what you need to stay afloat. People whom you've considered strong allies in the past may not be the best choices to support you now.

Changes in the dynamics of a relationship— whether it's a friendship, a love affair, or a workplace connection—can cause fallout that ranges from subtle to huge. Some folks will remain right by your side, unfazed by the changes that your illness brings about. Others will run screaming from the room, spurred on by their own sets of reasons—not knowing what to say to you, not knowing how to deal with your new limitations, or my personal favorite: fear that whatever you've got, it might be contagious.

The Rules Have Changed

At first, you may have to ask for help without much clarity about what you need. When your body hurts, it's difficult to do anything other than react—especially when you're in the grip of fear and uncertainty. You may erroneously project the judgments and opinions you hold about your situation onto others, inadvertently making false assessments. You may hide out for fear that people won't understand or see you in the same way. You may tough it out, never letting people know what you're going through, and ultimately compromise your health.

If you've gone through life as a giver, asking for and receiving help may be the hardest thing you've ever done. If you've had to call on people for assistance in the past, you may feel uncomfortable asking for help again.

I remember all too well how embarrassed I felt about my need to always be mindful of the relative proximity—and vacancy—of the nearest bathroom at work... how I dreaded telling my managers and co-workers that reliable Joan had to take a disability leave. It was a little easier at home—except when it came to my son.

He was 7 when my symptoms started and 20 when I went into full remission, and I felt incredibly guilty when I had to stay in bed for days at a time. When, during his teenage years, he seemed disinterested in my illness, I assumed his apathy was a protective mechanism to mask his anger at my not "being there" for him. Now that I'm writing this, I realize I really don't know for certain. Perhaps it's finally time to ask.

So, how do you sort facts from feelings? How do you tell the difference between a guilt response and a truly negative impact on another person? How do you know if you're steeped in paranoia or if you're really being treated unfairly? Discovering the answers to these questions is a rare gift—one of the upsides, if you will, of living with autoimmune disease (AD). If you choose to act in your highest good, you get to grow and learn and fall and recover and learn some more. Eventually, you may be lucky enough to get in touch with a new core of strength and humanity within yourself and create partnerships with others that move you to the depth of your soul.

It may help to remember that many people on your team may serve different purposes, thereby causing no undue stress on any one individual. It might also help to keep in mind—even if you can't quite believe it yet—that those who choose to support you do so *because they want to.*

Support at Work

Let's start out with the basic purpose of employment from the employer's point of view. You're paid to execute certain tasks and oversee various projects. Ideally, you and your co-workers become a strong network of talented people who fulfill the mission of the company. To make the system work, you're relied on (and, boy, do we take that to heart!) to do your part. It's a logical expectation.

The American Disabilities Act (ADA) states that companies of a certain size (15 or more employees) are required to provide reasonable accommodations for anyone with a disability who can otherwise perform the duties of his or her position, unless it can be proven that to do so would cause undue financial hardship for the employer. However, the onus still falls firmly on you. D. Diane Smith, a certified rehabilitation counselor, asserts, "The ability to successfully negotiate with your employer—or manager, supervisor, or teammates—is somewhat dependent on your self-confidence, physical strength, and conviction (1)." I would add that some luck comes into play. You'll fare better with a good support network and a decent employer. If you are overwhelmed, stressed, afraid, and otherwise uncertain about your rights, you may have difficulty acting on your own behalf. But you must.

Your managers will need your help. You may be the first person to present this kind of challenge, and they will probably need your assistance to figure out how to accommodate your needs so that you can still get your work done. They may also need your guidance to educate co-workers who will be impacted by any changes in your workload. The more you can do to offer solutions, the easier it will be for them to help you. And, if you think about it, that's precisely the case with any problem—personal or work-related.

Building Your Support Team via Leadership

An article by Fernando Montenegro Torres entitled "Are Fortune 100 Companies Responsive to Chronically Ill Workers?" states that, according to the Partnership for Solutions—an initiative to improve the care and quality of life for those with chronic health issues—an analysis of Medical Expenditure Panel Survey data shows that 47% of adults ages 21 to 65 report having at least one chronic health condition (2). This is a staggering statistic! If it's true—and we have no reason to believe it isn't—we have a lot of company on our journey. Are many of these people suffering in silence, keeping their health problems to themselves? If so, speaking up and talking about *your* situation might free them from their self-imposed isolation. Who knows: your openness could end up having a positive effect on more individuals than you could possibly imagine. But for now, let's get back to you.

Your efforts to build a strong support team—and to have those difficult conversations with your co-workers and employers—will change your role to one of leadership. Although you may get scraped and bruised in the process, you'll also have the satisfaction of knowing that you did everything possible to help yourself. Actions such as this build self-esteem—and we can use all the self-esteem we can get. If it turns out that you're working for an inflexible employer, or the company simply can't accommodate your needs, or you really can't come up with a solution to get your job done, you might as well find that out now.

In generations past, people made it a point to keep their work lives completely separate from their personal lives. Nowadays, the workplace often serves as the framework for a social network. Whether or not this is a healthy dynamic, it is a fact of life in the twenty-first century—and might even work in your favor. Allies are more easily developed when you have already established yourself as a competent, likable member of the team. What's more, if you have developed strong connections with the people you work with—and then neglect to let them know until it's too late that life has changed for you—you risk alienating the very same people you have been calling co-workers and friends.

For her 2005 article, "Factors That Influence Workplace Success," Rosalind conducted a survey of 50 people to get their input on the need for a support network (3). There was overwhelming agreement that "you need to develop allies to weather the periods when symptoms become worse or completely disabling." Furthermore, the survey revealed that 100% of those interviewed disclosed their chronic illness to at least one person at work. This suggests that it's really possible—and preferable—to open up to others in the workplace. Instead of toughing it out until you collapse, engaging in carefully planned and well-delivered communications can make you and your team stronger.

Seeking Outside Assistance

If you don't feel that you have the strength, understanding, or clarity you need to negotiate with your employer, start by building your external support network. It's much easier to fight on your own behalf if you are bolstered by people with some understanding of your situation. See the sidebar for some options to consider.

The Role Of Your Healthcare Team

When you live with AD, your doctors and other healthcare providers play key roles in helping you manage your life and your illness (for the sake of simplicity, I'll

Options to Consider

Some options you might consider that can help you garner support, education, and fortitude:

- Nonprofit organizations devoted to supporting persons affected by a specific illness. Many of them have local chapters; this is especially true if you live in or near a major city.

- Online blogs and bulletin boards started by people sharing similar health challenges.

- Person-to-person connections with other women in the same situation. Make sure to stay away from whiners. You're looking for people who strive to turn lemons into lemonade—and have had some success in doing so.

- Your physician's office. Your doctor probably has some good suggestions on where you might go to get the support you need.

- Members of your personal network who may have connections to resources you're not aware of.

- Professional therapists. They can help you sort through your emotions and feelings, clearing

(continued)

out the cobwebs of guilt and unnecessary fear that could hamper your ability to make good decisions and act in your own best interest.

- A professional coach. A coach can help you review your goals and objectives, assist you in formulating plans that effectively address the most pressing issues, and guide you to explore your options.
- Hospital support groups. These are created for people with various illnesses and usually hold their meetings right at the hospital.
- Vocational rehabilitation support services. These include, but are not limited to, private vocational rehabilitation counselors or state vocational rehabilitation services for their client-assistant programs.
- The Job Accommodation Network (www.jan. wvu.edu), a service of the U.S. Department of Labor (DOL) Office of Disability Employment Policy
- Searchable Online Accommodation Resource (SOAR) (www.jan.wvu.edu/soar)

use the words doctor and medical professionals to represent the entire spectrum of people who assist with your health). With the right people on your healthcare team, it will be easier to deal with the challenges that you face both personally and professionally.

Choosing the best people for these jobs can positively impact you in several ways. In addition to medical services, this portion of the team can also:

- Create a relative sense of certainty in the face of a very uncertain situation
- Give you the peace of mind that you have knowledgeable partners with whom you can have an honest dialogue
- Help you make good choices about the specific health-related issues that arise at work
- Provide access to resources and specialists as particular needs arise
- Educate you about the latest developments in research pertaining to your illness
- Partner with you to make the hard decisions regarding your work responsibilities, keeping you aware of when it's time to take a much-needed disability leave
- Provide a paper trail of your history that will help make a case for a medical leave

What's more, you can reasonably expect the medical professionals on your team to:

- Show openness and interest in alternative opinions
- Display caring, compassionate, nonjudgmental qualities and treat you with respect
- Work in harmony with the rest of your healthcare team
- See the doctor–patient relationship as a part nership
- Respect your concerns and accept your decisions, even when they may not agree with them

It's not always easy—nor is it as difficult as you might think—for you to be an active partner in these relationships and surround yourself with the people who suit you best. Remember—you're hiring these professionals to help care for you. Gone are the days when doctors were seen as definitive authority figures, and the patient's role was to follow blindly. In this Information Age, patients take a more proactive stance, whether it's regarding their course of treatment or their choice of healthcare provider. Trusting your instincts regarding the doctors assigned to you is as important as choosing your employers and personal friends. This is another important way in which you can act as the leader of your care, a warrior for your well-being.

You might have the wrong people on your health-care team if:

- You minimize your symptoms to your doctor because you don't want her to think you're complaining.
- The doctor shows impatience with your questions and concerns.
- The doctor's attitude is "It's my way or the highway."
- The doctor has a bedside manner that rubs you the wrong way.
- You have nagging feelings that the doctor is not giving you the best treatment or is failing to look at the entire picture.
- The support staff turns over frequently.
- You trust the members of the support staff more than the doctor.

I've had both great medical care and questionable medical care. All of my doctors have been good at what they do, but they were not always good for me. One doctor, with whom I had a positive relationship for a long time, became unexpectedly and unreasonably impatient with me during a colonoscopy. I was in pain during the procedure and was, apparently, making a lot of noise about it. I barely remembered what happened when I came out of anesthesia, but I was not ever fully comfortable with him afterwards. The experience did not fade, and I brought a lot of fear into my next colonoscopy two years later.

My original doctor had moved on, and his replacement was much more patient. This colonoscopy was pain-free and comfortable. I did my part, too—telling both the doctor and the nurses about my past experience, in the hope that it would not be repeated. I asked for careful monitoring of my anesthesia to make sure I was well sedated, and received assurance from the nurses—and a little extra hand-holding—to make it so.

When I moved a couple of years later, I had to put together another medical team. I asked my gastroenterologist for a referral, and confirmed that the new doctor accepted my medical insurance. He was reputed to be an expert in the field of gastroenterology and was involved on the board of the Crohn's and Colitis Foundation of America, so I felt good about the recommendation. I then found a primary care physician (PCP) in the same medical network (to comply with my HMO's referral requirements) who was reported to have some familiarity with Crohn's disease.

I discovered that the PCP didn't know all that much about Crohn's disease after all, and I began to realize that credentials do not tell the whole story. To complicate matters, I was having difficulty communicating with my new gastroenterologist. The deal breaker came on the day I attempted to discuss my concerns about azathioprine (Imuran), one of the medicines he'd prescribed. I'd take it for a little while and then stop. I'd go back to it again—and stop again. In the past, I was comfortable with the prescribed medications, but this one is an immune-system suppressant, and I was concerned about its long-term effects. Rather than listening openly to my concerns, he became argumentative. He insisted that Imuran was the only way to go, telling me that people have been taking it for years with no long-term side effects. Yada, yada, yada. He may have been right, but he was not acting in partnership with me. Fired!

I switched to another PCP who had direct experience with Crohn's disease. His sister lives with the disease, so he had both a professional and personal perspective. He recommended the doctor who is my current gastroenterologist—a much better doctor for me. He knows that the treatments he recommends are the best the medical profession has come up with to date, and he admits that much is still to be learned.

He has no issue with the complementary healthcare personnel I've added to my team, and his medical staff is involved in clinical trials, so they're aware of the latest developments.

When all is said and done, it's the consultative, respectful way he interacts with me that scores the true win. And, are you ready for a laugh? I'm taking the same medicines the last guy recommended! The difference? My current doctor allowed me to air my concerns, and he engaged in a respectful dialogue to help me sort it out until I felt comfortable with his recommendation. Since I've been in remission, we've lowered the dosage of Imuran and the frequency of my infliximab (Remicade) infusions from six times a year to four. That's another plus in my book. It's not all about the meds.

Are You on Your Support Team?

Building a support team starts with you. If you're going to ask for help from others, you must be prepared to do your part, as well. Some of the following behaviors and practices are often called up for review and examination in women with an AD.

Work/Life Balance

I can't even begin to express how important rest is. When your immune system is compromised, you are weaker. When your body is fighting day after day to heal itself, you need more R&R. There are no ifs, ands, or buts about it. If you're used to working all hours of the day and having all the energy you need, the realization of your limitations can come as quite a shock.

The first few months after I was diagnosed with Crohn's disease, I was convinced I could conquer my illness by sheer will. I will always remember driving around Southern California in the company van between bookstore locations, resting on the steering wheel (you can do that in vans) on California 60. I had Enya on in the background to help keep me centered. Truthfully, driving in the van between store locations was preferable to standing all day and walking up and down the aisles to help customers, shelve books, and the like. But I'm pretty sure that the California Highway Patrol would not consider California 60 to be a rest stop for the chronically ill. I really should have asked to be relieved of my duties as acting district manager and gone to half-time as a store manager. Oh, the power of denial!

And Enya? I hate that album. Although it's certainly not her fault, her music serves as a reminder of a time when I did not love my life.

During the workday, you need to find ways to slow down, stay centered, and conserve your energy. Take short breaks, and be sure to let the people around you know what you're doing. Use your lunch time to sit quietly, read, or take a nap—just get away from your desk.

Simplify your evenings by eliminating all unnecessary business activities, and figure out nontaxing ways to contribute to family time. Keep in mind that sitting quietly and comfortably while listening to your children and/or husband and/or significant other is a great way to participate. It's not necessarily about the things you do. Simply being and loving are huge acts of giving, probably ones that we should all—healthy or otherwise—engage in more often.

One of my colleagues who has been living with a variety of fluctuating symptoms of illness on and off since her early 20's, reluctantly pulls back on her involvement with our coaching chapter when her symptoms require she do so. She truly prefers to be able to attend our meetings as she enjoys the interactions with our community, but she's learned that she has to pull back and put her body first. For a while, she became involved with a project at the national level that allowed her to connect with other coaches around the country by phone and email, something she could more easily manage. She's been back to attend meetings this year, but declined a leadership position for now, knowing that the additional responsibilities might work against her health.

Boundaries

You are the authority on what works in your life and what doesn't. If you're not yet an expert at setting boundaries, your illness presents you with a great opportunity to learn this valuable practice. Setting boundaries is about creating limits with yourself and the people around you. It requires you to become aware of the things, feelings, and behaviors in your life that aggravate your symptoms and those that help you feel better.

Setting boundaries is a grown-up practice. Learning to live with the ups and downs of an autoimmune illness is a growing-up experience. They seem to go hand in hand.

So, how might this setting of boundaries play out? If you seek assistance from your doctor or any member of your team and are treated in a way that doesn't sit well with you, you have two choices. If you want to keep this person on your team, you need to address the issues that cause you concern. If this individual's style or approach consistently fails to work for you, walk away and look for help from someone else.

Nutrition

Nutrition is important for all bodies, but is especially critical for the body that needs to heal. Unfortunately, many of us with AD find that our bodies and eating don't always mix well. Our systems may be irritated by certain foods, our appetites may disappear completely, our digestive and nervous systems may be compromised by the medicines we take. We may even want to eat, but weakness and symptoms make it difficult.

Women with Crohn's disease and ulcerative colitis can have a very hard time keeping food down. Those with rheumatoid arthritis and fibromyalgia may have to severely change their diets if food sensitivities aggravate symptoms. Whereas you may have been free to eat what you wanted in the past, you may now have to work really hard to get the nutrition you so greatly need.

Nutrition may be one of the most difficult areas to normalize. There are probably as many recommended regimens as there are doctors and nutritionists. To be sure, many lay people are out there advocating nutritional programs and supplements that they're convinced will "cure" you. This is where discernment becomes especially important.

Shortly after my diagnosis, I met up with a natural doctor who tested me for all sorts of allergies. At the time, my symptoms were aggravated by eating, and I started to view food as an enemy rather than a friend. He told me I had to stop eating many foods that were a normal part of my diet. I searched through health food stores for items that this natural doctor recommended, and I often came up empty-handed. I had no appetite for them, and I was afraid. I was eating less and less and losing weight—while still working full-time and bearing the responsibility of caring for my son.

Two months later, I was admitted to the hospital after my first colonoscopy. It left me feeling weaker and sicker, so I called the doctor that evening. He told me that my colon looked like a train wreck, and he was pretty surprised I was functioning. I entered the hospital 10 pounds lighter (I was only 115 at normal weight, so I had very little wiggle room), severely anemic, and in lots of pain. During my 10-day stay, I barely avoided a blood transfusion, was put on a liquid diet, and received lipids intravenously to get my weight back up quickly. I was also introduced to Ensure, a liquid food supplement filled with vitamins and absent of dairy products. Ensure has since become one of my dietary friends when my symptoms dampen my appetite and compromise my intestinal system.

Clearly, you must do your part to improve the quality of your life when you are facing the challenges of an AD. As you move forward, don't lose sight of the fact that doing your part also means surrounding yourself with professional and personal allies who give you the care, support, nurturing, and understanding you need. John Donne said, "No man [or woman] is an island." The Beatles said, "I get by with a little help from my friends." And Rosalind and I say, "All you have to do is ask, girlfriend. The right team is out there—just waiting for your call."

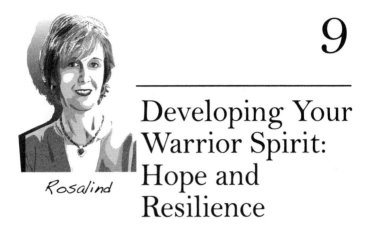

Rosalind

9

Developing Your Warrior Spirit: Hope and Resilience

My friend Janie had been going full throttle for months, putting all her efforts into building her business and caring for her three children. She describes it as "running on empty." She hasn't been watching what she eats, she hasn't been working out at the gym, and she skipped her yearly physical. She's always tired, and knows that she needs more sleep.

But Janie isn't worried. In a few months, she'll take a 2-week vacation and recoup. The way she tells it, "I've always lived with the assumption that a car should maintain itself. I found out I was dead wrong one day when my car came to a slow halt in the street. I remember looking at the gas gauge, and it was empty. I honestly never thought it could happen! Lucky for me, it was a short walk to a gas station. But I didn't learn my lesson.

"To this day, I rarely fill up until the tank registers close to empty. I figure there'll always be a gas station nearby. I guess I live my life that way, too."

As I listen to Janie (and feel like shaking her), I remember that she isn't like me—and probably isn't like you, either. She's not a member of this sisterhood. Thus far, at the age of 45, Janie can manage to keep going without stalling because she's always been healthy. She can refuel when necessary with little effort. She's willing to take herself to her limits, and her body makes only minor protests. She lives in a constant state of hope, because, at this point in her life, she can trust her body not to let her down.

But we, in the autoimmune disease (AD) sisterhood, can't afford to operate on a low gas tank. From quarter-full to empty is a slippery slope, and that can be very scary. Even if we once had the kind of hyper-resilience that Janie has, it's no longer part of our repertoire. It takes a lot more energy and time to recover when we get weary or sick.

Are you afraid that if you get run down you won't bounce back, so you choose to withdraw rather than pursue a life worth living? Did you skip that dinner party, opt out of that dream vacation, reject the big project that's coming up at work, order online rather than leave the house to go the mall? This kind of behavior isn't rare and, as a form of self-care, it's not necessarily bad. But this, too, is a slippery slope—the fine line between tending to your needs and allowing your life to grind to a halt.

I know it isn't easy. When considering the question *How much is too much?*, the answer can be pretty elusive. Too many variables get in the way on a moment-to-moment basis. That's why we need to master hope and resilience.

Hope is the belief in your ability to recover from whatever has knocked you down on any given day. *Resilience* is the ability to recover from the punch and land on your feet, or on your butt, or whatever supports you at the time. To cultivate your physical resilience, you must have the mental resilience that comes from a place called hope.

Living with hope does not mean ignoring your negative emotions, such as fear and anxiety. Instead, it's being able to counterbalance them to allow the positive, life-affirming emotions to bubble to the surface and thrive.

In his book, *The Anatomy of Hope*, Dr. Jerome Groopman devotes more than 200 pages to discussing hope and how it relates to illness (1). He describes what he considers to be two intertwined components of hope—intellect and feeling—which influence each other. He also makes a critical distinction between false hope and true hope.

False hope ignores the data, so we make decisions based on wishful thinking—a house of cards. True hope embraces the whole picture, allowing us to recognize that bad things do happen while looking for the best route to travel. Rather than obscuring the picture, hope heightens the areas of light.

Some people use their rational mind to achieve a state of positive emotions, while others cannot reach that place through cognition. For them, it's a purely emotional experience. No matter how you get there, each of us must reclaim a state of hope when faced with deep loss, such as the death of a loved one or a devastating chronic illness. And that requires resilience, defined by Groopman as "the maintenance of high levels of positive feelings and well-being in the face of significant adversity."

I know that I have found hope in the strangest of places. Before I became sick with multiple sclerosis, I struggled a lot—with everything. My own definition of myself was that I had to work hard for things, and there were many disappointments along the way. I felt sorry for myself, and no one would have described me as an optimist.

When I became very sick, I found that, for the first time in my life, something had happened to me for which I wasn't responsible. That took a tremendous load off my shoulders, allowing me to step back and say, "Wow, this has happened to me, but it's not *because of me*. The only thing I can do anything about, the only thing I have power over, is the way I think about it and respond to it."

In fact, that was the start of a 30-year journey that marked a new beginning of feeling enormous responsibility for all that I do—in the best sense of the words. How did it happen? I discovered a place called "hope."

Popular media will tell us that this attitude will make us healthier. I don't know about that, but I do know that hope makes it more possible to lead a satisfying life in the face of living with AD.

And the DNA of resilience? Will scientists discover that over the next decades? Perhaps. In the meantime, I've learned from my own experience, Joan's experience, and the stories of my clients that we don't have to be born with hope and resilience. We can develop our capacity for envisioning these qualities and our competence in developing and strengthening them.

So, what does it all mean for you? You can start by working on your own place called hope, and then developing whatever it takes for you to roll with the punches and get back up again. Joan and I think that the warrior spirit will allow you to be wise, take risks, and take care of yourself at the same time.

Finally, neither Joan nor I want to leave you with the impression that we believe illness is a blessing. My own life has been filled with joys and good fortune, but I wouldn't count living with chronic illnesses as one of them. On the other hand, I feel blessed that I have grown and gained wisdom from this experience. And I am a stronger person for it.

As long as AD has given you this opportunity, use it. Learn from it. And capitalize on it. Believe that you can influence what happens to you, even if you can't control it. Most important, grab hold of yourself and know that the one thing you can control is your own behavior. It's not a sprint—it's a marathon. And you can win it.

Keep working (at it), girlfriend.

Additional Reading

Far too many books are available on the subject of chronic illness and personal growth to cite them all here. Add to that the numerous disease associations, Web sites, and other resources, and it becomes an impossible task to create a comprehensive list. Instead, we've chosen to include only those we refer to in our narrative (and those that are our favorites).

Backstrom, Gayle. *I'd Rather Be Working, A Step-by-Step Guide to Financial Self Support for People with Chronic Illness.* New York: AMACOM, 2002.

Baron-Faust, Rita and Jill P. Buyon. *The Autoimmune Connection.* New York: McGraw-Hill, 2004.

Beaty, Joy E. and Rosalind Joffe. "An Overlooked Dimension of Diversity: The Career Effects of Chronic Illness," *Organizational Dynamics,* Vol. 35, No. 2. New York: Elsevier, 2006.

Bennetts, Leslie. *The Feminine Mistake: Are We Giving Up Too Much?*. New York: HyperionVoice, 2007.

Bridges, William. *Transitions: Making Sense of Life's Changes.* New York: Addison-Wesley, 1996.

Cornell, Ann Weiser and Barbara McGavin. *The Radical Acceptance of Everything.* Berkeley CA: Calluna Press, 2005.

Edwards, Paul and Sarah and Laura Clampitt Douglas. *Getting Business to Come to You.* New York: Tarcher, 1998.

Edwards, Paul and Sarah and Lisa M. Roberts. *The Entrepreneurial Parent.* New York: Tarcher/Putnam, 2002.

Groopman, Jerome. *The Anatomy of Hope.* New York: Random House, 2004.

Hayden, C.J. Get Clients Now!, 2nd ed. New York: AMACOM, 2007.

Horan, James T. Jr. *The One Page Business Plan.* Berkeley CA: The One Page Business Plan Company, 2004.

Jaff, Jennifer C. *Know Your Rights: A Handbook for Patients with Chronic Illness.* Farmington CT: Advocacy for Patients, 2005.

Klaus, Peggy. *Brag!: The Art of Tooting Your Own Horn without Blowing It.* New York: Warner Business Books, 2003.

Pitzele, Sefra Kobrin. *We Are Not Alone: Learning to Live with Chronic Illness.* New York: Workman Publishing, 1986.

Kubler-Ross, Elizabeth and David Kessler. *On Grief and Grieving: Finding the Meaning of Grief through the Five Stages of Grieving.* New York: Scribner, 2005.

Lahita, Robert G. *Women and Autoimmune Disease: The Mysterious Ways Your Body Betrays Itself.* New York: Regan Books, 2004.

Lazare, Aaron. *On Apology.* New York: Oxford University Press, 2005.

Matoushek, Nicole. *Acquired Hope: A Journey of Advanced Recovery and Empowerment.* Charleston SC: Booksurge Publishing, 2007.

Page, Martyn, ed. *The Human Body.* New York: DK Publishing, 2001.

Reichheld, Frederick with Thomas Teal. *The Loyalty Effect.* Boston: Harvard Business School Press, 1996.

References

If you'd like to read more about living and working with autoimmune disease, this is a chapter-by-chapter list of the source material for this book.

Chapter 1

1. Crohn's and Colitis Foundation of America. *The Crohn's Disease and Ulcerative Colitis Fact Book.* New York: John Wiley & Sons, 1983.

Chapter 2

1. Bennetts, Leslie. *The Feminine Mistake: Are We Giving Up Too Much?.* New York: Hyperion Voice, 2007.
2. Roberts, Sam. "51% of Women Are Now Living without a Spouse." *The New York Times,* January 17, 2007.
3. *Ibid.*
4. Partnership for Solutions, http://www.partner-shipforsolutions.org/statistics/prevalence.html.
5. National Organization on Disability, http://www.nod.org/index.cfm?fuseaction=Page.view Page&pageId=13.

6. Waddell, Gordon and A. Kim Burton. *Ils Work Good for Your Health and Well-Being?* London: The Stationery Office, 2006.

7. Clingerman, Evelyn, Alexa Stuifbergen, and Heather Becker. "The Influence of Resources on Perceived Functional Limitations among Women with Multiple Sclerosis. *Journal of Neuroscience Nursing* 2004; 36(6): 312–321.

8. Hobfoll, S.E. "Conservation of Resources: A New Attempt at Conceptualizing Stress." *The American Psychologist* 1989; 44(3):513–524.

9. Kralik, D. "The Quest for Ordinariness: Transition Experienced by Midlife Women Living with Chronic Illness." *Journal of Advanced Nursing* 2002; 39(2): 146–154.

Chapter 3

1. Beaty, J.E. "Chronic Illness Disclosure in the Workplace." Doctoral dissertation; Organizational Studies Department, Carroll School of Management, Boston College, 2004.

Chapter 4

1. Reichheld, Frederick (with Thomas Teal). *The Loyalty Effect.* Boston: Harvard Business School Press, 1996.

2. Super, Donald E. "A Life-Span, Life-Space Approach to Career Development." *Journal of Vocational Behavior* 1980; 16(3): 282–296.

3. Lahita, Robert. *Women and Autoimmune Disease: The Mysterious Ways Your Body Betrays Itself.* New York: Regan Books, 2004.

Chapter 5

1. Lazare, Aaron. *On Apology.* New York: Oxford University Press, 2005.

Chapter 7

1. Tieger Paul D. and Barbara Barron-Tieger. *Do What You Are*, 4th ed. New York: Little, Brown, 2001.
2. Edwards, Paul and Sarah and Lisa Roberts. *The Entrepreneurial Parent: How to Earn Your Living from Home and Still Enjoy Your Family, Your Life and Your Work.* New York: Penguin Putnam, 2002.
3. Ibid.
4. Klaus, Peggy. *Brag!: The Art of Tooting Your Own Horn without Blowing It.* New York: Warner Business Books, 2003.
5. Edwards, Paul and Sarah, with Laura Clampitt Douglas. *Getting Business to Come to You.* New York: Tarcher, 1998.
6. Horan, James T. Jr. *The One Page Business Plan.* Berkeley CA: The One Page Business Plan Company, 2004.
7. Hayden, C.J. *Get Clients Now!*, 2nd ed. New York: AMACOM, 2007.

Chapter 8

1. Personal communication.
2. Fernando Montenegro Torres, Fernando, et al. "Are Fortune 100 Companies Responsive to

Chronically Ill Workers?" *Health Affairs* 2001; 20(4): 209–219.

3.   Joffe, Rosalind. "7 Factors That Influence Workplace Success." Available at http://www.cicoach. com.

Chapter 9

1.   Groopman, Jerome. *The Anatomy of Hope.* New York: Random House, 2004.

Index